Health Care UK Spring 2001

The King's Fund review of health policy

Edited by John Appleby and Anthony Harrison

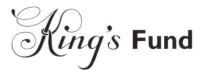

Published by
King's Fund Publishing
11–13 Cavendish Square
London W1G 0AN

© King's Fund 2001

First published 2001

ISBN 1 85717 436 4

A CIP catalogue record for this book is
available from the British Library

Available from:

King's Fund Bookshop
11–13 Cavendish Square
London
W1G 0AN

Tel: 020 7307 2591
Fax: 020 7307 2801

Printed and bound in Great Britain

*Cover image: Minuche Mazumdar Farrar
and Department of Health*

CONTENTS

POLICY ANALYSIS

DATASCAN

CONTRIBUTORS

John Appleby
Director, Health Systems Programme, King's Fund

Seán Boyle
Visiting Senior Research Fellow, London School of Economics

Chris Deeming
Research Officer, Health Systems Programme, King's Fund

Anna Dixon
European Observatory on Health Care Systems, London School of Economics and Political Science

Carl Emmerson
Programme Co-ordinator, Institute for Fiscal Studies

Jon Ford
Head, Health Policy and Economic Research, British Medical Association

Christine Frayne
Research Economist, Institute for Fiscal Studies

Stephen Gillam
Director, Primary Care Programme, King's Fund

Alissa Goodman
Senior Research Economist, Institute for Fiscal Studies

Anthony Harrison
Senior Fellow, Health Systems Programme, King's Fund

Justin Keen
Professor of Health Politics and Information Management, University of Leeds

Liisa Kurunmäki
Lecturer in Accounting, London School of Economics and Political Science

Richard Lewis
Visiting Fellow, Primary Care Programme, King's Fund

Peter Miller
Professor of Management Accounting, London School of Economics and Political Science

Ian Mocroft
Independent Consultant for Fiscal Studies

Elias Mossialos
Co-Director, LSE Health and Social Care, London School of Economics and Political Science

Bill New
Independent Health Policy Analyst

Cathy Pharoah
Director of Research, Charities Aid Foundation

Rebecca Shaw
Research Fellow, Centre for Health Economics, University of York

Peter Smith
Professor of Economics, Centre for Health Economics, University of York

In this issue

The BMA's review of health care funding ... health inequalities and weighted capitation ... charitable funding in health care ... long-term care ... health care spending in Europe

John Appleby

Money is always an issue in health care; there's never enough, it's spent on the wrong things, and when we look over the fence we see that our European neighbours seem to be more concerned about spending too much rather than too little! Of course, for a newly arrived Turkish immigrant in Germany or a child in a poor *arrondissement* in north Paris, total health care spending matters less than how it is shared out.

In this issue of *Health Care UK* we look at different aspects of health care funding – from alternative ways to raise money, to new developments in allocating it within the system and, of course,

attempts to pin down how much to spend in the first place.

The BMA has spent the last year gathering the public's and experts' views on alternative ways of funding the NHS. Its report was published earlier this year, and **Jon Ford** describes the main findings.

One alternative is to encourage more people to take out private medical insurance. Could this relieve some burden from the NHS? And how much would it cost? **Carl Emmerson, Christine Frayne** and **Alissa Goodman** from the Institute for Fiscal Studies explore the economics of such a tax break.

Having raised money for health care – by whatever means – there is the question of how it is shared out. Ever since the mid-1970s and the Resource Allocation Working Party (RAWP), the UK has been a leader in developing methods to share money across the country on the basis of need. RAWP and its successor, weighted capitation, aimed to tackle variations in access to health care. But now an additional objective is being considered – tackling variations in avoidable health inequalities. As **Rebecca Shaw** and **Peter Smith** note, this is a very laudable aim but more thought needs to be given to the details.

Further into the allocation process is the way money finds its way to general practitioners. **Richard Lewis** and **Stephen Gillam** raise a host of questions concerning the introduction of personal medical service (PMS) agreements – which started in 1998. Over the next four years, the majority of GPs are expected to take up this new contract. Lewis and Gillam reveal some early findings from research into the original pilots of PMS.

The NHS is not the only significant health care player. The tradition of charitable funding for health care continues, and **Cathy Pharoah** and **Ian Mocroft** describe the findings of a survey looking at this source of money in London.

Charitable funding also features in **Anthony Harrison**'s and **Bill New**'s article on health-related R&D spending. They find that publicly-financed R&D expenditure represents just over 11 per cent of the total amount spent on R&D.

Over the last few years it has been fashionable to compare the state of the UK's health care system with our European neighbours'. The comparisons, it has to be said, are usually unfavourable. But more than this, they are often wrong – or at least out of date in terms of developments in other countries' health systems. To rectify this, **Anna Dixon** and **Elias Mossialos** from the European Observatory (based at the London School of Economics) provide an up-to-date round-up of what's happening in a number of western European countries with regard to funding.

Meanwhile, back in the UK, **Liisa Kurunmäki**, **Peter Miller** and **Justin Keen** examine the financial flexibilities offered by Section 31 of the Health Act 1999. Although they say it is still early days, they note that there are growing numbers of examples of innovative joint-working arrangements involving the pooling of budgets between the NHS and social services. However, there is still a long way to go, and while the Health Act removes some structural hurdles to partnership working, effort, co-operation and understanding are still required to exploit the potential of the new flexibilities.

Despite the Government's response to the Royal Commission on long-term care financing, there is still concern that the issue of fairness remains unresolved. **Chris Deeming** and **Justin Keen** recast the long-term care debate in terms of equity and conclude that the Government's position and that of the minority report from two of the members of the Royal Commission are inconsistent.

Finally, **John Appleby** and **Seán Boyle** update their work examining the feasibility of the Prime Minister's 'aspiration' to raise UK health care funding as a proportion of it's GDP up to the level of the European Union average. Their conclusion is that the UK will still lag behind the rest of the EU as there is a rising trend in spending across the Union.

The BMA funding review

Jon Ford

For many years the BMA has been concerned at the apparently large and widening gap between the resources available for health care and the demands and needs of the population. Successive governments have struggled to find the resources to provide a service that is both comprehensive and universal. They have settled instead for one that treats expressed demand where possible and uses primary care, waiting lists and clinical judgement as regulatory mechanisms. The notion that the health service is comprehensive and free at the point of use has been preserved in spite of explicit evidence to the contrary. The maintenance of and increases in the real level of prescription charges, together with the progressive withdrawal of NHS dental and ophthalmic care, provide ample testimony to this. Add to this the increasing realisation that the service is under-utilised by those in the most socially deprived groups and it is clear that universality is also an illusion.

The substantial funding increases announced during 1999 and 2000 were seen by many, not least the Government itself, as the end of the funding debate. The country had seemingly got both the increases necessary and a guarantee that these would be maintained. Indeed, more than this it had the Government's 'aspiration' that such increases would continue until such time as this country spent as much on health as its European counterparts. Although we welcomed the extra funding and the political commitment it represented, we considered that the problems facing the NHS were more fundamental and needed more robust long-term solutions. We therefore initiated a review of health care funding, bringing on board representatives of patients, other professions and the private health care sector (*see box*). The outcome of the review was a report and supporting documents published on 6 February.[1]

The BMA has been associated with a number of joint initiatives in the past[2] aimed both at increasing resources and ensuring that such increases are sustained

PARTICIPATING ORGANISATIONS
The Academy of Medical Royal Colleges
The Association of the British Pharmaceutical Industry
The Association of Community Health Councils of England and Wales
The British Medical Association
BUPA
The Patients Association
The Royal College of Nursing
The Royal Pharmaceutical Society of Great Britain

within a stable funding environment, but this was the first time that so wide a grouping had been assembled to look at the topic.

The review posed four questions:

- what kind of health care does the public expect, want or need?
- what resources are required to provide this?
- can these resources be reasonably expected to be provided under present or alternative funding arrange-ments?
- what mechanisms can be used to bridge any 'affordability gap' that may emerge?

We commissioned public opinion research, both qualitative and quantitative, to assist with the first question and this was supplemented by desk research and a number of seminars at which patient groups were encouraged to give their views. The evidence from this part of the exercise and from the existing literature was simultaneously both surprising and unsurprising: unsurprising because it pointed to a high level of satisfaction with the NHS and its staff, albeit with some concerns about quality and delivery; surprising in that it pointed up major gaps in provision and a fundamental belief in equity in relation to health care. This last finding suggested early on in the process that proposals for radical change in the system of funding as against its level were unlikely to result from the review. Most proposals of this sort would not fill these gaps and would lead to a reduction in perceived equity.

Public opinion favours a health service that is

Public opinion favours a health service that is essentially free at the point of use and which aims to provide equal access to the same standard of care for all. However, there is a growing awareness that these principles are under great strain…

essentially free at the point of use and which aims to provide equal access to the same standard of care for all. However, there is a growing awareness that these principles are under great strain and inherently difficult to reconcile with a limited budget. Public support for the NHS as a concept is therefore balanced by a more pragmatic approach at the individual level. The gaps in provision identified by the public opinion and allied desk research fell into two categories – unmet need and unmet demand. The former is expressed by under-utilisation of health care resources in certain programmes by the most deprived populations. Unmet demand is not only illustrated by waiting lists for in-patient treatment; it is also evident in lack of access to services and treatments in areas such as mental health. Patient representatives gave us many examples of this. It is tempting for governments to act only on the most obvious measures of unmet demand – those associated with waiting for treatment.

However, the other gaps thrown up by the review are of as much, arguably even more, importance.

When we took evidence from those working in the service, three important financial issues were brought to our attention. First, we were told that the sums of money made available under the Comprehensive Spending Review, and subsequently, were of limited use to the service since they were earmarked or 'badged'. They were associated with new initiatives and targets at a time when general weighted capitation allocations were what were really needed. Second, we were told that, contrary to government protestations, the underlying deficits in Trust finances were genuine deficits, largely expressed as creditor balances and as such would have first call on any increased resources. Third, we were informed that the supposition that a large organisation such as the NHS was inherently inefficient was also wrong. Our attention was drawn specifically to the efficiency savings made each year for over a decade and to evidence put to the Health Committee that differences in Trust reference costs were not significant statistically.

When we set out on this exercise, there were two areas that many commentators felt would dominate the debate. These were the low level (in European terms) of private health spending in the UK and the extent of misuse of the service due to its being largely free at the point of use. The former would, it was supposed, lead to the search for mechanisms that would increase private funding levels, possibly even to wholesale reorganisation of the NHS along insurance or market lines. The latter would inevitably prompt calls for the introduction or extension of charges with the twin aims of improving funding levels and deterring demand. As already noted, however, the emphasis of the review was on patients' views. The extent to which these favoured equity meant that neither of these courses was a viable route for the review. Nevertheless, we looked in detail at alternative and complementary funding arrangements and received a small number of submissions that called for change of this kind.

Public support for equity was echoed in the views of clinicians. Seventy-two per cent of doctors surveyed as part of the review rejected

the view that universality had had its day in the NHS. Against this, 91 per cent felt that some sort of rationing in the NHS is inevitable. Doctors were drawing a distinction between a service that is universal and one that is comprehensive – a distinction we encountered repeatedly during the review. The conclusions we took from this were significant. At present, treatment is denied in the NHS on grounds of clinical effectiveness or cost effectiveness. Those who pass these tests may still have to wait for treatment but it is not denied to them. If the service is to reach out to those whose needs are at present not met or to those groups whose demand though expressed is ignored, this situation will need to change. The NHS will need to prioritise more explicitly and deny treatment more readily. That this will lead to a greater contribution from private medicine is both inevitable and inequitable. However, in arguing for equity in the publicly-funded service, patients are fully aware that those who can will buy treatment elsewhere.

The review's conclusions were summarised as follows:

The amount of money that can, and should, be spent on health care is to some extent a political decision, although it is also defined partly by public attitudes to taxation and public confidence in the process of government spending. Because demand cannot be accurately quantified, and because resources used in different ways will have different results, it is impossible to define the 'right' level of funding. *The NHS Plan* demonstrates that significant funding increases are both politically possible and, if not allocated carefully, limited in their usefulness. Although an essential precondition to improving services, increased resources alone can never be a complete solution.

The experience of other countries suggests that the problem of increasing demand and cost is widespread, whatever the means of funding. Introducing new funding mechanisms would bring new problems and inefficiencies, and would be no more successful than the current system in resolving the end-of-life costs and unmet need that represent much of the gap between demand and resources. Evidence suggests that people want to see more money spent on improving the health service in general, rather than on their own individual treatment. This concept of mutuality, or pooling of risk, appears to be central to what the public wants, and an essential element of an effective health care system. On grounds of both equity and efficiency, retaining a centrally tax-funded system that remains essentially free at the point of use is preferable to introducing other systems.

However, the concept of the NHS as a comprehensive service may have outlived its usefulness. It will be increasingly commonplace to see treatments that are judged to be of limited clinical effectiveness, not cost-effective or an inappropriate use of public funds, excluded from this system. The role of the private sector in meeting demands for these and other treatments will inevitably grow in importance, particularly in the self-pay sector as patients seek specific treatments that are explicitly excluded from the NHS. This growth should be encouraged and facilitated, although tax or other fiscal incentives would be an inequitable and inefficient means of doing so.

There are those who will be critical of the review in that it has not come up with a magic solution or number. Experience suggests that such approaches are overly simplistic and that explicit targets are invariably shown to be insufficient. The 1987 project, for example, concluded that health spending should keep pace with economic growth, with additional provision for catastrophic events (AIDS was one example). If, in addition, productivity improvements were maintained at the level of the service sector as a whole, then the demands on the system imposed by demography, technology and desirable service developments could be met. Although much of this has come to pass, it is evident that the system is still under strain.

REFERENCES

1. Health Policy and Economic Research Unit. *Health care funding review.* London: British Medical Association, 2001. (Full report and annexes on www.bma.org.uk)
2. See for example, O'Higgins M. *Health Spending – A way to sustainable growth.* London: IHSM, 1987.

Allocating health care resources to reduce health inequalities

Rebecca Shaw and Peter Smith

The massive injection of funds implied by the *NHS Plan* has stolen headlines. However, the Plan also implies another revolution in the financing of UK health care. For about 25 years the NHS has sought to allocate resources between geographical areas on the basis of securing equal opportunity of access for equal need. This basis for allocating resources is now under review, and ministers have adopted a new criterion: 'contributing to the reduction in avoidable health inequalities'. *The NHS Plan* states that 'by 2003, following the review of the existing weighted capitation formula used to distribute NHS funding, reducing inequalities will be a key criterion for allocating NHS resources to different parts of the country' (para 13.9). Although the new criterion superficially suggests similar broad aims

to that of securing equity of access, it actually signals a fundamental change of approach, which has profound implications for performance management as well as resource allocation. The purpose of this article is to give a commentary on some of the more important issues it gives rise to.

RESOURCE ALLOCATION

The NHS has in many respects led the world in the development of scientific resource allocation mechanisms. It started with the seminal work of the Resource Allocation Working Party (RAWP) in 1976, which sought for the first time to allocate NHS resources to regions on the basis of relative need rather than historical accident.[1] The criterion they adopted was to secure equal opportunity of access to patients in equal need, regardless of

where they lived. Although broadly successful in securing major shifts in expenditure over a period of 15 years, the RAWP system was always vulnerable to the criticism that it was not based on firm empirical evidence. However, a series of methodological reviews led to the development of the empirically-based York indices of health care needs, which were first implemented in 1995.[2] These indices, which reflect the equity of access criterion, continue to form the basis for the bulk of the financial allocations to health authorities in England.[3]

However, for the first time, allocations in financial year 2001/02 contain an element that seeks to address the new criterion of contributing to the reduction in avoidable health inequalities.[4] This 'health inequalities adjustment' (HIA) comprises £130 million targeted at those health authorities that are judged to be making the biggest contribution to current health inequalities. At first glance, this seems a very small amount when viewed in the light of the £37 billion distributed to health authorities on the traditional 'equity of access' criterion. In fact, £70 million is formally the HIA, with £60 million allocated to current Health Action Zone (HAZ) sites. However, as we note below, it marks a major departure from conventional resource allocation, and is likely to grow in importance in the future.

lifestyle, genetic and environmental considerations. There is considerable evidence that many populations suffering poor health outcomes suffer on all three counts: they use poor quality services, to which they have relative difficulty securing access, and they suffer multiple 'external'

Poor quality services for disadvantaged populations are in principle strictly a performance management (rather than resource allocation) issue. The right amount of money is being spent on such populations, but it is not being spent wisely.

spent on such populations, but it is not being spent wisely. The policy implication is that the quality defects should be rectified by (possibly radical) managerial action, but that extra resources are not the principal source of the problem. Therefore, there is no need for any major change to the resource allocation system. Rather, attention should be directed at securing high quality *management* of resources in deprived areas.

Poor access for disadvantaged populations implies that they are not receiving some services to which the remainder of the population secures access – that is, there is 'unmet need' amongst such populations. This compromises the validity of existing resource allocation formulae, such as the York indices (*see Box 1*), which are based on empirical links between need and utilisation. By definition, such indices will not capture any unmet elements of need. There will, therefore, be a need both for supplementary

REDUCING HEALTH INEQUALITIES

From the perspective of the NHS, it is helpful to think of avoidable health inequalities as arising from three broad sources: variations in the quality of NHS services; variations in access to NHS services; and variations in factors outside the control of the NHS, such as wealth,

disadvantage. However, the reason for considering the causes separately is that they have quite different implications for resource allocation and performance management.

Poor quality services for disadvantaged populations are in principle strictly a performance management (rather than resource allocation) issue. The right amount of money is being resource allocations outside of the usual formulae (to reflect the unmet need), and for performance management mechanisms (to ensure that the extra allocations are spent on the intended target: rectifying previously unmet need).

Poor life chances amongst disadvantaged populations pose the most fundamental challenge to the NHS. Health inequalities can arise from lifetime exposure to numerous sources, such as genetic, environmental, income, lifestyle, welfare service, and health utilisation variations. However, for capitation purposes, it is necessary to identify the specific potential contribution of *health care* to health improvement. If the NHS is to tackle health inequalities arising from this source, it will need to target the vulnerable populations in a way that it has not done hitherto. This might entail offering such populations preferential access to NHS services, in the form perhaps of accelerated access to surgery, or provision of therapies not available to all users of the NHS. In short, addressing health inequalities may require abandonment of the principle of equal access for equal *clinical* need, in favour of equal access for

some concept of equal *social* need. In some ways, this implies that resources allocated under the new criterion will supersede and formalise the philosophy of Health Action Zones, with its implied 'positive discrimination' in favour of deprived areas.

POLICY IMPLICATIONS

Under the traditional resource allocation criterion, there has already developed a wide range of *per capita* allocations. For example, in response to variations in need, as measured by the York indices, Manchester Health Authority receives 63 per cent more funding than West Surrey, and even bigger variations exist amongst Primary Care Groups and Trusts. Yet the health outcomes between the two health authorities are inversely related to such funding, with Manchester's under-75 standardised mortality rate standing at 135.4, compared to 79.5 in West Surrey. The new health inequalities adjustment means that – in order to address inequalities – Manchester receives £4.4 million in addition to the £408 million received through traditional criteria, whilst West Surrey receives no additional funding. The big questions are: to what

extent can such extra NHS resources affect health outcomes? And how much more are ministers prepared to widen the funding gap in order to make an impact on such large health inequalities?

Broadly speaking, the potential NHS interventions to address inequalities might take any one of the following forms:

- increased levels of treatment for targeted populations
- different forms of treatment
- earlier treatment
- more effective treatment (for example, making greater efforts to secure compliance)
- health promotion and education for relevant individuals and organisations
- co-ordination of other relevant agencies
- supply and analysis of improved information.

Without some indication of what specific action is required to address an inequality, the health services may fail to respond to the new policy objective in an effective way, implying that there is a need to indicate *how* the changes in capitation payments should be directed. Evidence from the Health Action Zones

BOX 1: THE YORK INDICES OF HEALTH CARE NEEDS

The principal methods for distributing NHS funds to health authorities have been developed at the University of York over the last seven years. The two original York needs indices related to acute services (£16.4 billion in 1999–2000) and in-patient psychiatric services (£3.4 billion).

The indices were developed using advanced empirical methods, and sought to determine the link between in-patient utilisation and social and economic conditions, after adjusting for demography, and taking account of certain variations in NHS supply. The indices capture the national average NHS response to need in the form of in-patient activity, and therefore cannot capture any 'unmet' need.

The acute sector index contains five variables:

- proportion of people of pensionable age living alone
- proportion of dependants living in single-carer households
- proportion of economically active people who are unemployed
- standardised limiting long-standing illness ratio for ages 0–74
- standardised mortality ratio for ages 0–74.

Other indices have a similar format. Further details can be found in the following references:

Carr-Hill R A, Sheldon T A, Smith P, Martin S, Peacock S, Hardman G. Allocating resources to health authorities: development of methods for small area analysis of use of inpatient services. *BMJ* 1994; 309: 1046–49.
Smith P, Sheldon T A, Carr-Hill R A, Martin S, Peacock S, Hardman G. Allocating resources to health authorities: results and policy implications of small area analysis of use of inpatient services. *BMJ* 1994; 309: 1050–54.
Rice N, Dixon P, Lloyd D, Roberts D. *Derivation of a needs based capitation formula for allocating prescribing budgets.* York: Centre for Health Economics, University of York, 1999.
Smith P, Rice N, Carr-Hill R. Capitation funding in the public sector. *Journal of the Royal Statistical Society* Series A.

and the emerging National Service Frameworks offers a potentially valuable resource in this respect. However, there is in general remarkably little reliable research evidence on 'what works' to reduce health inequalities.[5,6] Any new health inequality intervention should in principle be evaluated in order to ensure that it is effective (i.e. brings about the anticipated improvements in health) and cost-effective (i.e. brings about greater benefits for the money spent than alternative uses for society's scarce resources). However, this principle is not easily applied to interventions where the desired outcome is not simply an overall improvement but the narrowing of a health gap. An intervention that is effective in general public health terms may not reduce (indeed may exacerbate) health inequalities. (For instance, health promotion strategies focusing on individual health behaviours are more commonly and more quickly taken up by those with better personal and local resources. Thus, although there has been an overall reduction in the prevalence of smoking in Britain, there has been a widening gap between social classes in both the prevalence of smoking and smoking-related diseases.)

As we argue elsewhere, the volume of NHS funds to be directed towards the reduction of health inequalities also depends crucially on public preferences, and is therefore ultimately a political issue.[7] We have undertaken preliminary research on the importance attached by the public to the reduction of health inequalities, and have confirmed that a significant proportion of the population does consider the issue to be a policy priority.[8] However, we have found that the strength of opinion depends on the source of the inequality – for example, people appear to consider addressing inequalities arising from environmental causes, such as accidents, to be a more urgent priority than addressing inequalities that

result from individual behaviour, such as smoking. And there is a sizeable minority of the population that does not consider the reduction of any inequality to be a priority if it diverts resources from treatment based purely on a concept of clinical need.

Determining the sum to be devoted by the NHS to tackling an inequality is, therefore, not straightforward, as we must consider both its 'avoidability' (by the NHS) and its political importance. At present, ministers are in both respects flying blind, and the relatively small initial sum directed at reducing inequalities suggests an understandably cautious approach in the first year of operating the new criterion. However, as evidence begins to emerge, we would expect to see the size of the health inequalities adjustment to increase.

IMPLEMENTATION AND EVALUATION

In principle, implementing appropriate resource allocation mechanisms for the health inequalities adjustment requires the resolution of the following issues:

- identification of effective health care interventions designed to reduce the health inequality
- identification of disadvantaged groups at which the intervention will be directed
- identification of the areas where such groups live
- allocation of resources according to the group composition of an area
- ensuring that the resources are spent appropriately on the disadvantaged groups and the necessary interventions.

In its first year of operation, however, the distribution of the health inequalities adjustment has been based simply on the magnitude of an area's 'avoidable mortality'. This is defined as the number of years of life lost in the area under the age of 75 over a three-year period, where diagnosis of death is in certain broad categories deemed to be 'avoidable'.

This preliminary index is clearly chosen because of the ready availability of mortality data, and its plausible link to the sentiments of health inequality policy. However, it is clearly very broad-brush. For example, should all years of life lost be counted equally? Why use age 75 as the benchmark? Are the chosen diagnoses the most appropriate? Is current mortality (backward-looking, and the result of decades of experience) a suitable index of current need for inequality interventions (which are forward-looking)? How should migration be accommodated? These questions reflect the same sort of issues that troubled commentators on the original RAWP formulae, and led to their eventual replacement with more evidence-based indices. We would, therefore, expect that the current rough-and-ready index will in time be superseded by more sensitive indices of need, and are reassured to see that the Department of Health has put in place exploratory research to that end.[9]

As noted above, the new equity criterion also poses profound challenges for performance management. By definition, it implies that the NHS is not currently directing adequate resources towards populations that suffer health inequalities. The expectation must be that NHS organisations in receipt of health inequalities finance will use those resources specifically to address health inequalities. It will be surprising, therefore, if ministers do not scrutinise quite carefully the use to which such allocations are put.

Finally, the new resource allocation criterion also has profound implications for issues beyond resource allocation and performance management. The NHS will be anxious to seek out practical examples of strategies that have succeeded in reducing health inequalities. Yet, as noted above, the research base is very thin in this area, and there is a pressing need to evaluate rigorously the health impact of policies. The design of clinical trials may also have to be rethought, as there will be a need to know not only 'what works', but also what works for what types of patient, as defined (say) by life expectancy. The National Institute for Clinical Excellence may find itself having to formulate guidance, which suggests that patients with poor health expectancy may be offered treatment not available to healthier patients. And more ambitiously still, there remains a clear need to address the structured social inequalities that create health inequalities in the first place.[6]

The new health inequalities adjustment is a modest start, but does offer concrete hope of helping the NHS to start to address one of the most 'wicked' health policy problems: reducing health inequalities. To be successful it will require concerted action from all parts of the public sector, and not just the NHS, and it is likely in any case to take a long time to take effect. However, if properly implemented, the prize in time might be – for the first time in recent history – a concrete NHS influence on the reduction of health inequalities.

Shaw is funded by ESRC Grant L128251050. Smith is funded in part by the Department of Health.

REFERENCES

1. Department of Health and Social Security. *Sharing Resources for Health in England: Report of the Resource Allocation Working Party.* London: HMSO, 1976.
2. Smith P, Sheldon T A, Carr-Hill R A, Martin S, Peacock S, Hardman G. Allocating resources to health authorities: results and policy implications of small area analysis of use of inpatient services. *BMJ* 1994; 309: 1050–54.

3. NHS Executive. *HCHS revenue resource allocation to health authorities: weighted capitation formulas.* Leeds: NHS Executive, 1997.

4. Department of Health. *Health authority revenue resource limits 2001–02.* HSC 2000/034. London: Department of Health, 2000.

5. NHS Centre for Reviews and Dissemination. *Review of research on the effectiveness of health service interventions to reduce inequalities in health.* York: NHS Centre for Reviews and Dissemination, 1995.

6. Macintyre S, Chalmers I, Horton R, Smith R. Using evidence to inform health policy: case study. *BMJ* 2001; 322: 222–25.

7. Smith P, Shaw R, Hauck K. *Reducing avoidable inequalities in health: a new criterion for setting health care capitations.* York: Centre for Health Economics, University of York, 2000.

8. Dolan P, Shaw R, Smith P, Tsuchiya A, Williams A. *To maximise health or to reduce inequalities in health? Towards a social welfare function based on stated preference data.* York: Centre for Health Economics, University of York, 2000.

9. Department of Health 2001. Web site: www.doh.gov.uk/allocations/review.

CALENDAR OF EVENTS

AUGUST

1 **Professional regulation**: consultation documents published relating to the establishment of the Nursing and Midwifery Council and the Health Professions Council.

3 **Pathology**: £15 million allocated to the modernisation of pathology services supporting innovative projects at 23 demonstration sites.

7 **Public health**: in their first year of operation, NHS smoking cessation reported as having helped 6000 people to give up.

Waiting: teams from the Modernisation Agency sent into seven trusts that have experienced large increases in numbers of people waiting over 26 weeks.

8 **Winter planning**: increases in bed capacity announced, including 340 extra critical care beds and £63 million towards step-down facilities.

11 **Staffing**: NHS internet site announced, allowing all NHS vacancies to be advertised in one place by Spring 2001.

14 **Mental health**: £5 million allocated to services for children and adolescents with serious mental health problems, to be used for extra beds, specialist outreach services and new assessment procedures.

15 **Heart disease**: formation of ten fast-track teams to provide rapid responses for heart attack patients announced.

SEPTEMBER

6 **Winter planning**: plans announced for the Winter Emergency Services Team to visit 40 local health authorities to support winter planning.

Cancer: NHS prostate cancer research programme launched, leading to a fourfold increase in directly-commissioned research into prostate cancer.

7 **Hospitals**: Secretary of State urges hospitals to expand bed numbers and review all planned changes in the light of the bed projections in the *NHS Plan*.

8 **General practice**: new core contracts for GPs in personal medical services pilots announced, which will require them to:

- deliver patient access to a primary pare professional within 24 hours and a GP within 48 hours by 2004, though many expected to achieve this by 2002
- implement the standards set out in the cancer guidelines, and in the National Service Frameworks for coronary heart disease, mental health and in others to follow

- keep skills up to date by committing 30 hours a year to their personal and professional development
- undertake three clinical audits a year in the pilot, to drive up standards
- strengthen good employment practice in primary care, including an expectation that nurses in pilots will receive the full Pay Review Body recommendations.

11 **NHS Direct**: new computer system announced involving a seven-year partnership with Axa Assurance. It will become the standard for all NHS Direct nurses.

Drugs: Government welcomes European Commission on orphan drugs, which will provide incentives by waiving fees payable to the European Agency for the Evaluation of Medicinal Products and guarantee market exclusivity for ten years.

12 **NHS Plan**: *Pharmacy in the Future – implementing the NHS Plan* published. Key points of the National Plan for pharmacy include:

- by 2004, electronic prescriptions will be used routinely, with GPs e-mailing prescriptions directly to the pharmacist
- by 2004, patients will be able to get repeat prescriptions from their pharmacist without having to see their GP
- by 2002, any person in England who calls NHS Direct will be referred to their local pharmacist if appropriate
- 500 new one-stop primary care centres around the country, which will allow pharmacists to work alongside GPs, dentists, opticians, health visitors and social workers
- the improvement of out-of-hours pharmacy provision
- the establishment of an Action Team to promote better use of prescribed medicines.

18 **Pay**: Government evidence to Pay Review Bodies proposes that the NHS pay regime be reformed to address recruitment and retention difficulties, especially amongst nurses, reward those staff given greater powers under the *NHS Plan*, and ensure that consultants who make an exclusive commitment to the NHS get fast-track access to bonuses.

Dentistry: NHS Dental Strategy published. The main aims are:

- expanding the role of NHS Direct – using it as a gateway to all NHS dentistry by advising patients where they can find an NHS dentist
- ensuring that patients are given better information in the surgery, and investigating how to fund urgent out-of-hours NHS dental treatment
- investing up to £35 million in 2001–02 to modernise NHS dental practices and equipment, benefiting patients and dentists alike
- setting up a £4 million Dental Care Development Fund for immediate use, helping dentists to expand their practices and treat more patients
- introducing an £18 million fund for rewarding dentists who are committed to the NHS
- establishing up to 50 Dental Access Centres by April 2001

- encouraging new partnerships between the NHS and potential providers of dentistry, including independent organisations – giving patients reliable new sources of NHS dentistry.

20 **Critical care**: extra £15 million allocated to critical care services for children.

21 **Winter planning**: campaign launched to encourage greater take-up of flu jab.

Staff: recruitment campaign launched in London and south-east to encourage nurses and other staff to return to the NHS.

26 **Hospitals**: eight trusts to act as models of good practice for hospital cleanliness.

27 **NHS Plan**: memberships of the NHS Modernisation Board announced.

Cancer care: NHS Cancer Plan launched. This set out targets for treatment of urgently-referred patients, investment in equipment such as scanners, more nursing and medical specialists and the establishment of a National Cancer Institute.

Support services: compulsory market testing dropped. NHS Trusts and Primary Care Trusts will still need to demonstrate value for money. They will be required to measure themselves against the best the NHS can offer – including services operated by the private sector where services are already contracted out – to see whether or not they are meeting value for money and the high standards that are now required. If not, they should market-test the service, but with a new emphasis on satisfaction and quality, as well as cost.

Screening: national programme announced to detect thalassaemia and sickle-cell disease in pregnant women and newborns.

Heart disease: NICE guidance issues on super aspirins and mini-defibrillators, and major expansion of rapid access heart clinics announced.

OCTOBER

3 **Dentistry**: start of the commitment scheme for NHS dentists, which is designed to reward those working mainly within the NHS.

4 **Staff**: *Improving Working Lives Standard* published. It summarises the commitment expected from NHS employers to create well-managed, flexible working environments that support staff, promote their welfare and development, and respect their need to manage a healthy and productive balance between their work and their life outside work.

5 **Public health**: Government reaffirms intention to ban tobacco advertising following decision by European Court.

Neonatal care: £6.5 million announced for neonatal intensive care equipment.

Staff: further action announced to improve working conditions for junior doctors, including targets for working hours and standards of accommodation and catering.

Public health: projects launched to improve access to fruit and vegetables.

8 **Asthma**: NICE issues guidance on inhalers for children under five.

13 **Genetic testing**: the Genetics and Insurance Committee announces that the reliability of the genetic testing for Huntington's disease is sufficient for life insurance companies to use when assessing applications for life insurance.

16 **Hospitals**: new requirement brought in for hospitals to monitor levels of acquired infection from 1 April 2001, covering wound infection after orthopaedic surgery, bacterial bloodstream infections and infection becoming apparent after discharge.

17 **Winter planning**: appointment announced of 'change agents' – dedicated winter planners – to help local health economies prepare for winter.

Prescribing: electronic transmission of prescription pilots announced.

18 **NHS Direct**: NHS Direct information points launched in accessible public places, including universities, supermarkets, pharmacies and hospitals.

Staff: annual appraisals for consultants introduced, which are intended to identify where consultants need support in keeping up to date. In addition, a £40 million fund announced for the hardest working consultants.

19 **Commissioning**: new directions announced to require health authorities to carry out the decisions of regional specialised commissioning groups.

23 **Winter planning**: advertising campaign launched to inform people of the full range of health care options open to them during winter.

25 **Prescribing**: consultation paper published outlining options for extension of nurse prescribing, including:

- minor injuries and ailments like burns, cuts and hayfever
- promoting healthier lifestyles such as help with giving up smoking
- chronic disease management including asthma and diabetes
- palliative care

Staff: measures announced to recruit and retain Asian and minority ethnic staff.

31 **Out-of-hours services**: *Raising the Standards for Patients: new partnerships in out-of-hours care* published, setting out a new model for out-of-hours care. and encouraging further integration of GP services with NHS Direct and A&E departments.

Private sector: Secretary of State signs concordat with the private sector, covering elective care, critical care, intermediate care and workforce and service planning.

NOVEMBER

1 **NHS Plan**: presidents of the British Associations for orthopaedics, dermatologists and ear, nose and throat surgery announce their support for the 'Action On' programmes.

3 **Dentistry**: the location of 49 dental access centres and the allocation of the £4 million dental care development fund announced.

7 **Staffing**: plans announced to recruit Spanish nurses and refugee doctors.

9 **Fraud**: penalty charges of up to £100 introduced for those falsely claiming exemption from NHS charges.

14 **NHS Plan**: Cash allocations to health authorities for 2001–02 announced, an average increase of 8.5 per cent in cash terms over the previous year.

Hospital food: Loyd Grossman appointed to head a chef's panel to advise on a national NHS menu. Other improvements in food are planned. Nearly £40 million will be spent over the next four years to improve the quality and availability of hospital food for patients. The key elements are:

- by 2001, a 24-hour ward call service will provide patients with meals at any time of day or night, with a new NHS menu designed with the help of leading chefs. This 24-hour service will be available in all NHS hospitals
- by 2004, new 'ward housekeepers' will be in place in half of all hospitals to ensure that the quality, presentation and quantity of meals meets patient needs and that patients, particularly elderly people, receive appropriate meals when they require them
- a new national franchise for hospital catering will be looked at, to ensure that hospital food is provided by organisations with a national reputation for high quality and customer satisfaction
- patients will be consulted regularly on the quality of the food they receive, and there will be unannounced inspections of the quality of hospital food

- dieticians will advise and check on nutritional values in hospital food.

15 **Waiting lists**: second interim report of booked appointments programme published.

NHS staff: strategy published for improving the status, training, pay and career opportunities for the allied health professions.

Diet: the free fruit in schools pilot projects launched.

16 **Prescribing**: ambulance paramedics now allowed to use a wider range of injectable medicines to provide emergency treatment for those suffering a heart attack or other life-threatening conditions.

20 **NHS Direct**: NHS Direct prospectus launched setting out proposed developments in out-of-hours care.

21 **Drugs**: NICE issues new guidance for the use of Relenza for high-risk patients:

- those aged 65 or over
- those with chronic breathing diseases (including asthma) who need regular medication
- those with significant heart disease
- those with a weakened immune system
- those with diabetes

It recommends:

- drawing up agreements to enable pharmacists and nurses to supply Relenza, provided they are satisfied the patient needs it and meets the criteria. The Government recently introduced legislation to allow this to happen nurses fielding calls from patients who may need Relenza and making a recommendation to the GP on whether it should be prescribed or not. This will help cut down the number of GP consultations.

Clinical quality: CEPOD report *Then and Now* published, which compared findings in 1990 with 1998–99. It found that care had improved over that period, but 5 per cent of patients did not receive high dependency or intensive care post-operatively, for want of a bed.

22 **NHS Staff**: phase 2 of Positively Diverse launched after extensive piloting. The programme is intended to improve the working lives of staff and promote equality of opportunity.

27 **Staff**: new contract agreed for junior doctors, awarding large increases to those working over the 56-hour target, plus new accommodation and catering standards.

30 **Private sector**: concordat proposed for the care home sector to better manage capacity and provide better disability services.

DECEMBER

4 **Winter planning**: *NHS Winter Plan 2000–2001* published, involving:

- wider provision of flu vaccination for at-risk groups
- nationwide access to health advice through NHS Direct
- developments in primary, intermediate and community care
- 1350 more general and acute hospital beds and 445 more critical care beds
- increases in local authority

placements in nursing homes, intensive home care packages, and new intermediate care services.

5 **Cancer screening**: the programme extended to women aged 65 to 70.

8 **Purchasing**: National Specialist Commissioning Advisory Group annual report published. This includes an overview of regional specialised commissioning.

Public health: a research programme launched into mobile phones and the publication of two leaflets summarising the health evidence of mobile phone handsets launched.

12 **Commission for Health Improvement**: first three pilots of hospitals in Southampton, North Derbyshire and Sunderland published.

13 **Drugs**: fourth meeting of the Pharmaceutical Industry Competitiveness Task Force recommends:

- clarification of the rules and processes for prescribing medicines outside the NHS
- clearer definition of the current regulations to provide information to patients
- moves to secure effective industry involvement in the development and implementation of National Service Frameworks
- actions to make progress on all these issues were agreed.

14 **Health Action Zones**: nine employment pilots launched, including support for the New Deal programmes, help for single parents, development of work-related skills and occupational health.

18 **Pay**: the Government accepts the recommendations of the Pay Review Bodies of above-inflation increases for all NHS staff covered by them of at least 3.7 per cent and larger increases for senior nurses.

20 **NHS Plan**: *Implementation Programme* published. It sets out the national framework for implementation within which regional and local plans will fit. It will provide the framework for reviewing Health Improvement Plans (HImPs) and agreeing Service and Financial Frameworks (SaFFs), Joint Investment Plans (JIPs) and Primary Care Investment Plans (PCIPs) for 2001–02.

Mental health: proposals for reforming the Mental Health Act published. It is proposed that the new legislative framework will include a significant range of new safeguards. New legislation will introduce:

- a new independent tribunal to determine all longer-term use of compulsory powers
- a new right to independent advocacy
- new safeguards for people with long-term mental incapacity
- a new Commission for Mental Health
- a statutory requirement to develop care plans.

21 **NHS Plan**: Health and Social Care Bill published. The Bill provided for the abolition of community health councils, the extension of free nursing, new rules on the confidentiality of patient information, extension of prescribing right, and changes to the regulation of pharmaceutical services.

- **Drugs**: NICE publishes new guidance on Relenza, recommending its use for high-risk patients.

29 **Screening**: new programme for detecting hearing loss in babies announced.

JANUARY 2001

2 **Cancer care**: results of the Cancer Services Collaborative published, reporting large reductions in waiting times.

3 **Vaccination**: figures published showing that meningitis C has almost disappeared in the target groups following an extensive immunisation campaign.

4 **CJD**: £200 million allocated for NHS decontamination and sterilisation equipment.

5 **Pay**: ambulance workers, scientists and clerical and maintenance workers awarded pay increases of at least 3.7 per cent, with laboratory staff receiving further increases above that level.

Clinical standards: review of Harold Shipman's clinical practice published.

8 **Clinical quality**: *Assuring the Quality of Medical Practice*, guidance for implementing the proposals in *Supporting Doctors, Protecting Patients*, issued. It sets out the arrangements for setting up the National Clinical Assessment Authority.

12 **Vaccination**: the Committee on Safety of Medicines and the Joint Commission on Vaccination and Immunisation conclude that the triple MMR vaccine is 'very safe'.

15 **Neighbourhood renewal**: a National Strategic Action Plan published. In addition to the broad range of measures to improve health across the country, the Plan contains a series of commitments specifically aimed at improving health outcomes in deprived areas, including:

- the first ever national health inequalities target
- 200 extra Primary Medical Services Schemes by 2004
- modernisation of primary care premises in deprived areas to provide patients with better access to services
- free and nationally available translation and interpretation service to be available from every NHS premises through NHS Direct.

16 **General practice**: £30 million allocated for 2001–02 to improve access to GP practices and other local services, and extending the range of services that patients can access locally.

Telemedicine: British Library launches the Telemedicine Information Service.

17 **Hospitals**: a further £30 million allocated to improve standards of cleanliness, and ward sisters to receive authority from April 2000 to withhold payments from contractors if standards are not reached.

18 **NHS Plan**: Department of Health publishes *A Policy Position Statement and Consultation Document* on the 'traffic light' system proposed in the *NHS Plan*.

Cancer care: national cancer standards published, covering information, staffing, skill levels, communication and management.

Recruitment: campaign launched to bring midwives back into the NHS.

Hospitals: guidance issued on the prevention of hospital-acquired infections.

19 **Drugs**: NICE recommends that Aricept, Exelon and Reminyl should be made available to those with mild to moderate Alzheimer's disease and Rilutek for those with Motor Neurone Disease.

26 *Your Guide to the NHS* published, replacing the *Patient's Charter*.

30 **Organ Retention**: Report of Inquiry into Organ Retention at Royal Liverpool Children's Hospital, and announcement of establishment of Retained Organs Commission.

Wealthy and healthy: charitable funds in health provision today

Cathy Pharoah and Ian Mocroft

What is the role of charity in providing health in the twenty-first century? The establishment of the National Health Service was largely aimed at replacing a system of health care dependent on charity. But 50 years on, charity is still with us. In fact, growing public concern over levels of State health provision over the last decade has been accompanied by growing public acceptance of the contribution that both private and charitable funds can make.

The public is generous in its support of health – about £600 million is raised annually by the public for national medical and health-related charities. Health and medical support has been the fastest-growing charitable cause over the last 15 years, particularly attracting legacies from the public, which have constituted more than a quarter of charitable income. Equally significant sources of charitable funds for health-related causes are the grants provided by the huge corporate, private and hospital foundations, and more recently by the National Lottery.

NEED TO VALUE CHARITABLE GIFTS FOR HEALTH

Ever appreciative of their own health and medical care, people are clearly more than willing to give to these causes, regardless of any expectations they might have about what the State should provide. The Government has recently provided a stimulus for the giving of major gifts that health and medical causes and hospitals appear to be able to attract. From now on, the market value of gifts of quoted stocks and shares can be offset against income tax in the year in which the gifts are made. Such gifts are already exempt from capital gains tax, and so represent a double tax benefit to the potential donor. How can the philanthropic potential of an increasingly healthy and wealthy society best be fostered, and valued? How can we ensure that the charitable contribution is used to maximum effect and benefit?

In fact, there is almost no systematic information on charitable support in health, medical and related areas today. A first step towards valuing the role of charitable funds, therefore, is to obtain a picture of their extent and role. To begin to answer some of these questions, the King's Fund, together with Guy's and St Thomas' Charitable Foundation, jointly commissioned CAF (Charities Aid Foundation) to assess charitable funds in health in London, as a follow-up to previous CAF studies of the role of the voluntary sector in health provision. Although it was only possible within the limits of this particular project to look at London, the findings present an indication of national trends, partly because such a large proportion of NHS charitable funding itself is held in London.

SOURCES OF CHARITABLE FUNDS: AN INNOVATIVE STUDY

This study was both innovative and challenging, because of the many different sources of charitable funds for health. The NHS itself had £1.8 billion of charitable assets for the whole of the UK in 1999, producing a charitable income of £314 million. These funds are administered by over 500 trustee bodies. Charitable funding for health, however, comes from many sources other than the NHS's own funds. Major sources include the Wellcome Trust, which had an income of £307 million in 1999, PPP Healthcare Medical Trust, with an income of £25 million in 1999, and the King's Fund itself, with an income of £10.5 million in 1999. Other contributors

include the numerous independent grant-making charitable trusts, recently estimated by CAF to give about £178 million nationally to health (12 per cent of their funds), the National Lottery, commercial companies, Leagues of Friends, the general public and the non-profit or charitable hospitals and hospices that provide specific health services. As noted above, a great deal of health-related work is also supported by the many well-known health charities, such as Imperial Cancer Research Fund, Cancer Research Campaign, British Heart Foundation and special appeals such as Tommy's Campaign.

WHAT WAS INCLUDED AND EXCLUDED WITHIN THE DEFINITION OF 'HEALTH'?

To develop some overall estimates of health support, it was necessary to combine sensibly these very different kinds of charitable funds used in their very different ways. It was decided to include all activities that are similar or directly related to those provided by the National Health Service, including clinical and biomedical scientific research, education of staff, health policy and management studies, etc. Some activities carried out in universities associated with teaching hospitals, and broader philanthropic health purposes such as the maintenance of art collections belonging to a hospital, were also included. Services, or funding of services similar or equivalent to those of local councils' social services departments, however, were excluded. It was also recognised that to focus on services for Londoners involved some artificial distinctions because phil-anthropic funds spent in London have considerable national benefit, just as much of the research conducted outside London benefits the capital.

ALMOST HALF A BILLION FOR LONDON

Using these definitions, it was finally estimated that charitable funds for health, medical and related work in London totalled £473 million per annum. This considerable sum is equivalent to about 10 per cent of the NHS's own expenditure of £5 billion on services for people living in London in 1998–99.

Almost half of this sum consisted of grants from trusts and companies, whose support reached approximately £214 million for health in London. Half of this sum consisted of the charitable funds of the long-established teaching hospitals in inner London, who spent £107 million in 1998–99. It was estimated that the next largest source, the grant-making trusts, spent a further £81 million (including the London Livery Companies' charitable activity).

The remaining £259 million was spent in London by charities that provide direct services or raise money from the public to provide services or promote medical and medical-scientific research.

HOW ARE THE CHARITABLE FUNDS USED?

A pretty clear profile of spending was obtained, which revealed a heavy skew towards research and the needs of the acute hospitals, and a thin spread of support over other areas. Over half (51 per cent) of the £214 million spent by the grant-making charitable trusts went to clinical, biomedical and medical-scientific research. Buildings, equipment and other running costs accounted for a further one-fifth of the charitable grant-making – in this category more was spent on buildings than on equipment.

Outside of these three major categories, small proportions of funding were spent on community-based projects (6 per cent), in-patient welfare (5.5 per cent), staff welfare (5.2 per cent, largely on training and education of NHS staff) and other unspecified grants to NHS institutions at 4.9 per cent.

LACK OF DETAILED INFORMATION

Disappointingly, there was also nearly £19 million (8.7 per cent) of spending where little or no public information was readily available regarding how it was spent. In addition, there was rarely enough detail within the broad categories of research, patient welfare, etc, to develop an adequate picture of which particular areas benefit from charitable funds and consequently to assess where there might be unmet needs. There would be considerable benefit from better data collection.

CHARITABLE FUNDS UNDERPINNING RESEARCH

One major finding of the study, therefore, was the dependence of research on charitable funds. Funding of health-related and medical-scientific research, particularly in the large teaching hospitals and universities, was easily the largest category of expenditure by the grant-making trusts. However, a substantial proportion of fund-raising and service-providing charities' expenditure would also have gone to support such research (for example, the cancer research charities and other medical research bodies such as the British Heart Foundation).

This may not be a surprising conclusion in itself – the current distribution still reflects the history of London's medical services before the formation of the NHS, with each voluntary hospital having its own charitable fund, some of which were very rich and others less so. Moreover, research lies at the heart of the charitable objects of some of the charities included in the study. Nonetheless, the pattern of expenditure detailed in the study is largely historical, and a debate on how trustees can maximise the use of charitable funds for health benefit in London is long overdue. The governance of traditional 'hospital' charitable funds is being separated from the institutions in which they have traditionally been administered, and funds are now registered as independent charities with the Charity Commission. This gives trustees more scope and freedom in determining their use. Additional funding could be made available for many areas other than research and acute care that could make a difference to the health needs of Londoners.

CHARITABLE FUNDING TO MEET LONDON'S NEEDS

Few charitable sources pay particular attention to community-based projects. Exceptions include the King's Fund itself and the National Lottery Charities Board. Yet some of London's pressing health needs arise from the broader problems of poverty and deprivation, and from London's heterogeneous population, with its very diverse health experience. Such issues may gain little direct benefit from extra expenditure on traditional health provision; they need multi-disciplinary, community-based approaches. Charitable funders could pioneer these. It has also been argued that they could focus on more strategic interventions, influencing policy and pump-priming important changes with an ultimate impact several times greater than their own original inputs.

Many grant-makers have a policy of not funding health projects because they believe that health attracts sufficient funding from others, including government, but the figures in this study show that this is a misapprehension. The funding of health needs at the neighbourhood level is an integral part of tackling poverty, deprivation and marginalisation.

Those seeking charitable funds to extend the services for health and health-related sciences that they provide are clearly pushing against an open door. Greater awareness, information, and debate about the role of philanthropic funds in health could help to unlock even greater public generosity and support. Recent changes to tax relief on giving offer huge scope to those raising funds for health. For example, the health providers could help themselves by ensuring that their own employees have access to payroll-giving schemes in which donors can now make a gift of any size, tax free, direct from their pay. As an added incentive, the Government has pledged to add an extra 10 per cent to all donations made in this way for the next three years. Such schemes, added to the new tax relief on major gifts of shares, could make a significant impact on charitable funds for health.

For further information on this research contact Cathy Pharoah at CAF. For further information on tax-effective giving to charity, telephone CAF on 01732 520000.

The finance of research and development in health care

Anthony Harrison and Bill New

Since its foundation, the NHS has embodied, particularly through its teaching hospitals, a commitment to the promotion of clinical practice through the 'appliance of science'. Over the same period, the UK has developed a thriving and internationally competitive pharmaceutical industry, also research-based, which, along with its competitors, has made major contributions to the ability of the NHS, and other health services, to reduce the incidence of disease and to treat patients successfully.

In this paper, our prime focus is on the use of public funds to finance the NHS R&D programme and other health-related research paid for out of public funds. As we shall see, however, the public and the private roles are closely intertwined and must to some extent be considered together.

In Part 1 we set out the current pattern of spending from all sources and how it is financed. We find that publicly-financed expenditure represents only a modest fraction of the total budget allocated to research in this field.

In Part 2 we consider the attempts which have been made to improve the way that public sector funds are allocated. In Part 3 we look at a small number of general issues about the content and direction of the publicly-funded programmes, and finally in Part 4 we draw some general conclusions.

PART 1: HOW MUCH IS SPENT BY WHOM?

There is no one source for estimating total current spending on health-related R&D. In the mid-1990s, however, the House of Lords Select Committee on Science and Technology produced an estimate that distinguished six principal categories of expenditure on what they describe broadly as 'medical research'.[1] Five of these – less the Service Increment for Teaching and Research (SIFTR), the research element of which is now within the NHS R&D element – are set out in Table 1 and Figure 1.

Figure 1: Total spending on health care-related research and development (£m, most sectors 1996–97)

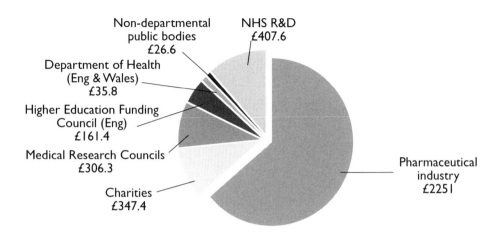

Non-departmental public bodies £26.6

NHS R&D £407.6

Department of Health (Eng & Wales) £35.8

Higher Education Funding Council (Eng) £161.4

Medical Research Councils £306.3

Charities £347.4

Pharmaceutical industry £2251

At the time the Committee produced its report, the scale of publicly-funded research spending within the NHS was unknown. Notionally, part of SIFTR 'paid for' such research, but there was no reliable means of determining how much went on R&D. A more or less arbitrary estimate of 25 per cent was made when the R element was taken into a separate funding stream and became the basis of the figure shown in the Table for NHS R&D.

As Table 1 and Figure 1 show, the private sector, particularly the pharmaceutical industry, is far the largest component of UK spending on medical research, carried out both in-house, but also through sponsoring work in universities, biotechnology companies and in NHS settings. The Association of the British Pharmaceutical Industry (ABPI) claims that pharmaceutical companies carry out almost 20 per cent of all industrial research and development in Britain,

spending more than 20 per cent of their gross output on R&D.

Table 1 also indicates that charities (ie. the not-for-profit sector) contribute a significant proportion of research funding, particularly for cancer. In total, in 1998–99, the amount of money from just two of the cancer charities – The Imperial Cancer Research Fund and the Cancer Research Campaign – was over £100 million, and as we shall see in this field, they fund more research than the public sector. The largest individual contributor is the Wellcome Trust, a medical charity that derives its funds from a single large endowment rather than from continuous voluntary giving and which is the only charity free to fund research in any field.

The principal and oldest public institution in the field of medical research is the Medical Research Council. It was originally set up as the Medical Research Committee in 1913, and was

Table 1: Total spending on health-related R&D

	UK (£ millions)	Year of data
Pharmaceutical industry[1]	**2251.0**	**1997**
Charities[2]	**347.4**[3]	**1998–99**
Wellcome Trust	172.9	
Imperial Cancer Research Fund	55.3	
Cancer Research Campaign	51.3	
British Heart Foundation	43.1	
Arthritis Research Campaign	16.8	
Leukaemia Research Fund	8.0	
Medical Research Council (UK; gross)	**306.3**	**1996–97**
'Intramural' (research units and institutes, etc.)	158.1	
Higher education institutions (through grants, etc.)	125.5	
Other (Government departments, research councils, private industry, local authorities, etc.)	16.0	
Overseas	6.7	
Higher Education Funding Council (England): Medical science	**161.4**	**1996–97**
Department of Health (England and Wales)	**35.8**	**1996–97**
Policy research programme	28.7	
Medical technologies (Medlink)	0.8	
Other research	4.5	
Radiation protection research	1.9	
Non-departmental public bodies	**26.6**	**1996–97**
Public Health Laboratory Services Board	6.0	
Centre for Applied Microbiological Research	5.8	
English National Board for N, M & HV	0.8	
UK Transplant Support Service Authority	0.2	
National Radiological Protection Board	4.1	
National Institute for Biological Standards and Control	4.2	
Health Education Authority	3.7	
Bio Products Laboratory	1.9	
NHS R&D	**407.6**	**1996–97**
R&D 'service support' for NHS providers	343.7	
NHS R&D programme	63.8	

1 from www.abpi.org.uk.
2 AMRC. *The Association of Medical Research Charities Handbook 2000*. London, 1999.
3 Top six total.
Note: The category 'Health Departments and NHS' is split into three sections following the Science, Engineering and Technology (SET) statistics 1998: all data from this source unless otherwise specified.

incorporated under its present title by Royal Charter in 1920. Its purpose, as set out in its Royal Charter, is:

- to encourage and support high-quality research with the aim of maintaining and improving human health
- to train skilled people, and to advance and disseminate knowledge and technology with the aim of meeting national needs in terms of health, quality of life and economic competitiveness
- to promote public engagement with medical research.

Like all research councils, the MRC pays for the research that it supports from a grant-in-aid through the Office of Science and Technology. It also receives funds for specific projects from other government sources.

Its function is to promote the balanced development of medical and related biological research in this country. It employs research staff directly at its own major research establishment, the National Institute for Medical Research at Mill Hill, and at 53 research units, most of which are close to or within a university or hospital but administered separately. In addition, the MRC funds research by means of a range of external grants, including administrative support for the Institute of Cancer Research and Strangeways Research Laboratory, a number of programme grants to support the long-term work of research departments, and project grants that are designed to provide support for a specific piece of work. Finally, it supports the training of researchers through fellowships and studentships. Table 2 sets out its main areas of work and the budgets attached to each.

In addition to the MRC, the Biotechnology and Biological Sciences Research Council spent £175 million in 1996–97, much of which will have implications for clinical work. For example, £24 million was spent on 'Genes and developmental biology', and £21.9 million on 'Biomolecular sciences'.

It should also be noted that the Economic and Social Research Council funds many projects that will be of interest to the management and organisation of NHS, although it is difficult to estimate how much of its overall spend for 1996–97 – £57.7million – is of relevance. One of the ESRC's subject areas, 'Lifespan, lifestyle and health' accounts for £4 million, but this certainly underestimates the total amount of NHS-relevant research in social science disciplines.

Table 2: MRC main areas of work, 1996/97

	£ million
- Macromolecules, cells & development biology	59.9
- Genetic blueprint & health	43.7
- Nutrition, chemicals, radiation & trauma	9.8
- Infections, immunity & inflammation	56.8
- Neurosciences & mental health	51.4
- Organs systems & cancer	40.6
- Health services & public health	15.4

The fourth main contributor, the Higher Education Funding Council, allocates its funding as a block grant and so it has been difficult to disentangle precisely how much is ultimately devoted to medical research. However, it was possible to make an estimate of the funding 'earned' by medical research by using the formula for establishing the research-related element of the block grant – which is based on research-active staff in each department combined with the department's performance in the most recent Research Assessment Exercise. This is 'QR' funding, which accounts for 95 per cent of all research funding. The House of Lords Select Committee estimated that about 20 per cent of QR was earned by medical subjects – 13 per cent by clinical and 7 per cent by non-clinical.

Since 1993–94, however, the OST SET statistics have separated out expenditure on five broad subject areas for HEFC-funded R&D and SET expenditure: natural science, medical science, engineering, social science and humanities. This offers a more convenient means of obtaining data for specifically medical research expenditure. Table 3 gives figures for 1996–97 for England.

It is difficult to establish precisely how much of this might be considered relevant to health care R&D, as some from social science and humanities and even engineering and natural sciences will contribute to health care, e.g. through the invention of medical devices or providing the basis of a broad understanding of some of the physical processes in the environment and elsewhere bearing on health.

Spending from the Department of Health can be separated into the Department's own research programme and those of various non-departmental public bodies on the one hand, and NHS R&D on the other.[2] The Department of Health's principal stream of research is the Policy Research Programme, which aims to provide a knowledge base for health services policy, social services policy and central policies directed at the health of the population as a whole. These include population studies of health and social well-being, lifestyle issues, promotion of health environmental factors, prevention, social care for adults and children, health service organisation, and strategies for care of patients with particular diseases or conditions (i.e. the National Frameworks).

Table 3: HEFC for England, research expenditure by broad discipline, 1996/97

	£ million
Natural science	224.5
Medical science	161.4
Engineering	148.3
Social science	159.0
Humanities	126.2

NHS R&D funding falls into two principal categories. First, it provides financial support for NHS providers for in-house research. It also covers 'excess' or 'service support' costs (not treatment or research costs) of research conducted in NHS providers for other bodies – and of relevance to the NHS – but funded from a variety of sources including research councils and charities.

Second, it finances R&D commissioned specifically on behalf of the NHS through national and regional programmes. These have now been re-cast from a large number of time-limited programmes into three programmes: Health Technology Assessment (HTA), Service Delivery and Organisation (SDO), and New and Emerging Applications of Technology (NEAT).

The HTA programme attempts to answer questions such as 'does this treatment work, at what cost and how does it compare with others?'; it is also developing more capacity to undertake 'fast-track' assessments, e.g. for NICE. The SDO programme aims to provide knowledge about how the organisation and delivery of services can be improved to increase the quality of patient care, ensure better strategic outcomes and contribute to improved health. NEAT exists to promote and support, through applied research, the use of new or emerging technologies to develop health care products, the main purpose being to overcome a development barrier and also a perceived 'funding gap'.

Over and above the figures included in Table 3, other parts of government also make contributions to health-related research, including the Department of Trade and Industry via its support for research in industry, the Office of National Statistics and the Scottish Executive.

As the above account indicates, it is difficult to link the flows of finance described in Table 1 to particular areas of research in anything other than a general way. However, at a detailed level, information is available in the National Research Register of ongoing and recently completed research projects funded by, or of interest to, the UK NHS. Information is held on nearly 70,000 projects, as Table 4 sets out.[3]

The Register is not comprehensive and, as far as we are aware, has never been analysed into areas or types of research. However, the figures are sufficient to indicate the scale, in terms of project numbers, of health-related research work in the UK.

PART 2: POLICY DEVELOPMENT

As the previous section has shown, the UK as a whole commits substantial resources to health-related research and development. Most of this is not under the direct control of government, but significant elements are the responsibility of the Department of Health, the Department for Education and Employment, and the Department of Trade and Industry (via the Office of Science and Technology). In this section we sketch out the developments in policy in recent years that have been aimed at improving the way the resources under direct public control are allocated.

However, because of the close links between this expenditure, the NHS and the other sources of funding, the way these resources are allocated has important implications for other research funders. As the figures set out overleaf

Table 4: Ongoing and recently completed health research projects (as at 2001)

Database	Number of projects
NRR Projects database	
Ongoing projects	22,107
Complete projects	46,350
MRC Clinical Trials directory	
Clinical trials	158
Register of Registers	
Registers of research	69
Registers of Reviews in Progress	
Ongoing reviews	318
Health Research at York database	
Research at the CHE and NHS CRD	129

indicate, the 'production' of research within the NHS is part of a complex system comprising within the NHS itself the provision of care and clinical teaching. Traditionally, the teaching hospital has been the locus where these three elements intersected. The NHS itself intersects with the universities, which are both producers of research and undergraduate medical teaching. Their funding also comes from several sources – the Department of Education, the research councils and the private and not-for-profit sector.

The private and not-for-profit sectors taken together command much larger budgets than all the public sources combined, and to a large degree they are independent of the public sector, able as they are to decide themselves how much they spend on what. But in key areas they are highly dependent on the public sector. Both require access to NHS patients, and in some cases NHS researchers and clinicians for scientific work, and above all clinical trials. To meet these needs, the NHS requires a physical and human infrastructure with

the necessary scientific and organisational skills to be in a position to work in effective collaboration with the private and not-for-profit sector, as well as with publicly-funded researchers. The same is true of the universities.

The way that the Department of Health and the NHS allocate funds to research both within and outside the NHS is therefore only part of a very complicated set of arrangements that underpin the production of health-related knowledge. In what follows, however, our main focus is on the way that public funds controlled by the Department of Health and the NHS are deployed.

As we saw in the previous section, health-related research has attracted funding from public sources since the First World War, when the predecessor of the Medical Research Council was founded. But it was only after the publication in 1988 of a House of Lords report,[4] the precursor of the one we drew on above, that a coherent policy began to emerge.

This report identified a series of failings in the then organisation and management of medical research; in particular, it concluded that:

> The NHS should be brought into the mainstream of medical research. It should articulate its research needs; it should assist in meeting those needs; and it should ensure that the fruits of research are systematically transferred into service. (para. 4.4–7)

In the first half of the 1990s, two main steps were taken to improve the way that finance for research was allocated. First, the development of a centrally-managed R&D programme within the Department of Health, and second, a reform of the way that finance within the NHS was allocated. We take these in turn.

The House of Lords 1988 report recommended that an independent organisation should be established to be responsible for most publicly-funded research. This proposal was not accepted by the Conservative Government. Instead, an R&D programme was established within the Department of Health; its aims were set out in *Research for Health*,[5] published in 1991.

The initiative led to the establishment of a machinery for determining research priorities overseen by the Central Research and Development Committee, a series of time-limited research committees charged with determining research priorities in particular areas, the development of regional programmes plus the centrally-directed programmes noted in section 1: the Health Technology Assessment Programme, the Policy Research Programme, the NEAT, and finally the Service Delivery and Organisation Programme launched in 2000 (having been promulgated in 1996).

In these ways, over a period of nearly ten years, machinery for determining priorities and directing resources towards them slowly took shape.

This process also required a change in the way that research was financed within the NHS. The immediate stimulus to change, however, was the introduction, following the 1991 NHS and Community Care Act, of the NHS internal market. This appeared to threaten the viability of the 'research trusts', whose costs were higher than average. Although, as noted above, they were supported by the 'R' element of the SIFTR, whether or not this was adequate was unclear.

A task force was set up under Professor Antony Culyer to 'consider whether to recommend changes in the conduct and support of research and development in and by the NHS, and if so to advise on alternative funding and support mechanisms for R&D'.[6]

The resulting report recommended (among many other things) the establishment of a levy system on all NHS providers, to be used for a variety of purposes (*see Box 1*). The levy was subsequently established and it is now used to fund both R&D within NHS providers and the NHS R&D programme.

It was envisaged at the time that the proceeds of the levy would be used to redirect research resources to areas of high priority. A special 'census' of research activity, carried out following the publication of the Task Force report, confirmed that these resources were then highly concentrated on a few hospital trusts. However, in practice, only limited shifts have occurred since the arrangements were introduced in 1998. The main beneficiaries of the funding

BOX 1: PURPOSE OF THE NHS R&D LEVY

To meet the costs of the NHS's contribution to the infrastructure and environment in which health and health services R&D can flourish and be well managed. This includes contributing to the training of people intending to pursue R&D as an integral part of their careers.

To contribute to the development of the capacity of the NHS and others, to identify needs for health and health services R&D, and to evaluate the costs and benefits of R&D.

To meet certain costs incurred by providers of NHS services in supporting non-commercial R&D activity paid for by funders external to the NHS (e.g. charities, research councils).

To allow providers of NHS services themselves to support, carry out or commission R&D of direct interest to the NHS.

To commission, on behalf of the NHS as a whole, specific R&D activities identified as national or regional priorities for the service.

To contribute to the dissemination of the findings of R&D.

To make a contribution to encouraging the use and exploitation of R&D findings, and the promotion of an evaluative and evidence-based culture in the policy and practice of the NHS, through the development and evaluation of techniques for implementing the results of R&D.

directed to providers remain the large teaching and research hospitals, despite the fact that in contrast to the early 1990s a large number of other providers do receive some funding.

In 1999, a strategic review of the workings of the levy[7] was published. This concluded that although a lot had been achieved following its introduction, further changes were needed. In particular:

- a clearer focus on NHS needs and priorities was needed
- improved quality assurance systems for research programmes were required
- there should be systematic involvement of wider health communities and consumers in NHS Research & Development; and

- research capacity in terms of research training and career prospects needed to be developed.

During 2000, the Department of Health published a series of consultation papers that took up and developed these themes and which foreshadow further reforms both of the way that priorities within publicly-financed research are determined and in the way that such research is financed.[8]

As far as funding is concerned, it is proposed to divide funding for NHS research within the 'service support' element of the budget (see Figure 1) into two streams:

NHS Priorities and Needs R&D Funding will address:

- the implementation of the NHS priorities in National Priorities Guidance
- the programme of National Service Frameworks and the National Performance Assessment Framework
- the work of the National Institute for Clinical Excellence, and
- the needs of the NHS in implementing Government policy. (para. 2.26)

NHS Support for Science will meet the NHS costs of supporting R&D under agreed standards of strategic direction and quality assurance by the research councils and other eligible R&D funding partners. It will include, where appropriate, an element for the costs of developing R&D proposals and for building work around that supported by the external funder.

The relationship between the new and the old arrangements is shown in Figure 1.

Figure 1: Components of NHS R&D funding

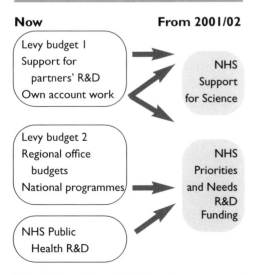

To support the new arrangement, the Department of Health is to 'provide leadership' by:

- publishing a Science and Technology Strategy in early 2001
- publishing a cross-government Public Health R&D Strategy in 2000, clarifying (amongst other things) the contribution of the NHS and its partners to public health R&D
- giving strategic direction to work supported by NHS Priorities and Needs R&D funding
- expressing NHS priorities and needs for research in these areas in dialogue with its partners.

The new system is due to be implemented during 2001–02. Accordingly, the existing system has been effectively put on hold, i.e. budgets were rolled forward until the new arrangements could be brought in. It will be some time, therefore, before substantial changes in the use of the levy funds can be made.

As this very condensed account indicates, the process begun in 1991 is far from complete and hence the core weaknesses of the situation as the House of Lords found it in 1998 have not yet been fully addressed. This is not to say that a great deal has not been achieved. The Strategic Review of the Levy concluded:

> 5. The implementation in 1997 of many of the recommendations of the 1994 report Supporting Research and Development in the NHS (the Culyer Report) initiated a revolution in research management in the NHS. In the few years since the Research & Development programme has been established every region and major hospital has research & development managed with explicit research and training programmes and plans for future development.

Achieving these changes is something with which the NHS can be justifiably proud.

Similarly, an outside observer, Nick Black,[9] also concluded that considerable progress had been made:

Although it is too soon to establish the value of the R&D program in any rigorous way, some interim assessment is justified, if only to attempt to influence its future direction. The program can be judged a success on several criteria. It has started to redress the balance between basic, clinical, and health services research in terms of funding; raised awareness of and concern for the outcome of health care among clinicians and managers; introduced much greater coherence and logic to research funding decisions; raised the profile and respectability of dissemination and implementation of scientific evidence; mobilized many scientists and clinicians who traditionally were not involved in health care R&D; and funded many research projects and training opportunities. Although none of these can be shown to have benefited the public directly yet, these achievements are necessary stepping stones to that goal. (p.503)

However, the Review also indicated that despite the fundamental changes that have been made since 1988, some of the basic issues identified then remain to be tackled effectively. The consultation papers and other documents appearing during 2000 represent a response to those findings. But as things stand, the system by which resources are allocated to R&D remains opaque both within the NHS and outside it and, as a result, it remains unclear just what the resources nominally devoted to research actually purchase.

A report by the Science and Technology Committee of the House of Commons, *Cancer Research: A Fresh Look*,[10] notes

'the conviction of many witnesses ... that most of the R&D funding was disappearing into general support for NHS hospitals and that little of it was actually made available for research purposes'. It found this situation 'deeply unsatisfactory'.

Similarly a research report[11] on the implementation of the Culyer reforms found that:

existing cost measurement and accounting systems have proved inadequate for the purpose of tracking and managing R&D support costs at the operational level.

In other words, some of the basic building blocks of an effective system of allocating finance to research within the NHS have yet to be put in place. As we shall see in the next section, some more fundamental issues are yet to be addressed.

PART 3: SOME GENERAL ISSUES ARISING

As the account above shows, the public funding of R&D is in a state of transition and it will be some time before the impact of the proposed changes can be judged. Despite the proliferation of documents relating to publicly-financed R&D, a number of issues have received very little attention. In this part we focus on a small number of these.

THE SIZE OF THE PROGRAMME

In 1991, *Research for Health* proposed that spending on research should rise to 1.5 per cent of the NHS budget over a period of five years.

To permit the development of the R&D programme, it is intended to move over a 5 year period to a target expenditure of 1.5% of the NHS budget. To put this in perspective, for the 1989/90 NHS budget for England, 1.5% would have amounted to £317 million, including NHS expenditure already allocated.

At that time the proportion was just under 1 per cent. That proportion rose during the 1990s but the original target was never met.

Curiously, none of the documents referred to above discuss whether or not it remains valid and if not what should replace it. With the recent substantial rise in the overall budget, the implication is that R&D should also receive a significant boost.

That initial target was, of course, largely aspirational; Sir Michael Peckham, the first Director of the Department of Health R & D programme, subsequently indicated to the House of Lords committee that it should not be regarded as a rigid target. At the time it was set, there was very little knowledge available about what was being spent, and how productive that spending was. Furthermore, the volume of work focused on trying to determine how productive research was, was also limited.

In essence, that remains true now. A number of projects designed to measure the value of research were funded during the 1990s, including a series of pilots carried out by the Health Economics Research Unit at Brunel University. But, as Buxton and Hanney have shown,[12] reviewing this and other work, the obstacles to achieving effective evaluation are severe. They concluded that:

It is certainly too early to answer the question as to whether the NHS R&D programme will give value for money, but it is possible to draw some conclusions, partly from analysis of research funded before the start of the NHS R&D programme. It has been possible to estimate the nature, and to a degree the extent, of payback from some past projects or programmes, particularly those aimed at particular policy issues. However, it has also been possible to identify projects that had virtually no payback. It is clear that good science is necessary but is not sufficient.

It is not surprising, therefore, that very little has been published by those responsible for NHS and other centrally-funded R&D as to the benefits that the programme as a whole has been realising. Nor is there, in the public domain at least, any indication of the technical merits of proposals that are not receiving funding (except in the case of cancer: *see Box 2*)

The absence of such evidence in itself does not demonstrate that the programme is large enough, or even too large. It may reflect more on the continuing problem – identified in the 1988 report, in the Culyer report and in the Levy review – of attracting and maintaining the supply of research, particularly in the areas where the level of research remains low, i.e. the organisation of delivery and service development. The Strategic Review of the Levy concluded that:

25. A major weakness in the present Research & Development programme is the shortage of experienced health service researchers in a well developed career structure. This shortage is a major threat to the Research & Development programme.

A start has been made to address these issues but it will be some time before effective action is taken. As things stand, therefore, it is arguable that difficulties with the supply of the necessary research skills are an effective constraint on how fast the programme can grow, particularly in the less well-established fields, even if a case could be made for expansion in them. We suggest below that a *prima facie* case for expansion in some areas can be made.

PRIVATE AND PUBLIC ROLES

As the figures set out in the first part of this paper indicate, the private and the not-for-profit sector together vastly outweigh spending from public sources. But despite the large amount of attention that publicly-financed R&D has attracted since 1991, the question of what the public and private roles should be has been rarely addressed and then only in a limited way. With rare exceptions, official papers describing the publicly-financed programme do not address the question of what the proper role of the public sector is, given the massive spending in the private sector.

The NHS has always largely relied on the private sector for the development of new drugs and medical devices while, as noted above, the private sector has relied on the NHS to assist with some areas of research and with the organisation of trials. This complementary relationship was endorsed in the *NHS Plan*, which set out a number of proposals for making the partnership between public and private sectors work better.

However, it did not go on to consider which areas of research into drugs and devices might be desirable from the viewpoint of the NHS and its users, but which the private sector might not wish to work in. That issue arose in the House of Lords inquiry into complementary medicine.[13]

The House of Lords inquiry into complementary medicine noted that spending within the R&D programme on complementary medicines was very limited. It was also limited within the 'industry' supplying medicines and treatments. Much of this industry is small scale and many of its products are not patentable. The Committee recommended 'that companies producing products used in CAM should invest more heavily in research and development'. (para. 7.81)

It noted, however, that there was no patent protection for most products in this area. Furthermore the research capacity does not exist. The Committee, therefore, made recommendations designed to create it within the public arena without specifying how this might service the commercial sector.

The same issue arises with so-called orphan drugs, i.e. drugs that serve a market too small for the private sector to consider investing in it. Here a policy response is in the process of being developed in the form of a European Directive that offers enhanced patent protection. However, that may not be enough. If so, there is an obvious case for public funding, as there may be for so-called alternative medicines.

Although the Department of Health acknowledges that the private sector 'uses the test-bed provided by the NHS to develop products', it does not appear to have considered the terms on which that support is offered at a strategic level, what the limits to that support might be and how these link with other elements of government policy, particularly licensing medicines and medical devices and the role of NICE.

In contrast, the Science and Technology Committee felt that the public role was far too small in cancer research and recommended a large increase in it (*see Box 2*). But it too did not set out a reasoned case for a particular balance between public and private finance.

THE COMPOSITION OF THE PUBLIC ROLE

As we have noted, the composition of the then pattern of spending was one of the key features singled out for criticism in the House of Lords 1988 report. Since then, there has been a vast amount of work designed to improve the composition of the research receiving funding (as well as its quality).

As we have noted, the NHS Central Research and Development Committee was established to provide a strategic framework for the programme and subsequently a large number of areas were reviewed. In 1995, formal arrangements were introduced to engage consumers in the determination of research priorities, and when the SDO programme was formally launched in 2000, an extensive 'listening exercise' was conducted resulting in the identification of ten areas of concern:

- organising health services around the needs of the patient
- user involvement
- continuity of care
- co-ordination/integration across organisations
- inter-professional working
- workforce issues
- relationship between organisational form, function and outcomes
- implications of the communications revolution
- use of resources, such as ways of disinvesting in services and managing demand

- implementation of major national policy initiatives such as the National Service Frameworks for coronary heart disease and mental health.

Furthermore, as National Service Frameworks areas develop, they are each identifying research needs for each service covered, and the consultation papers issued in 2000 promise that further attention will be given to the determination of priorities.

But, despite this activity, some areas continue to be neglected. We have argued elsewhere[14] that the R&D programme has persistently ignored certain types of problem.

The continuing emphasis on clinical issues in research priorities means that the issues identified in earlier chapters as critical to the running of the Service remain neglected. This neglect is not simply a matter of lack of resources; rather, it stems from a persistent failure to acknowledge the implications of the central and the local management role, in particular, the vast range of areas where clinical and other issues interrelate and can only be tackled by combining skills and disciplines. In other words, the needs of the NHS as a system of health care delivery have been neglected. (p.234)

The SDO programme represents an attempt to overcome this bias. But by the end of 2000 it had made only a small number of commissions and spending remained very low. Thus, very little has yet been done to shift the balance towards service delivery, i.e. away from research to development.

As Peckham has argued,[15] 'the prime orientation of R&D has been towards the first element research to the neglect of the second'. He concludes, therefore, that 'the requirements for health service development need to be separately defined and supported'.

He goes on to note that:

> The development task includes issues related to hospitals and other elements of the health care built environment, health service infrastructure, user and workforce questions, the design of health service processes and delivery systems, and the relationship between lay people and professional staff. The scope of development also encompasses issues such as clinical guidelines, quality and performance measures, as well as the criteria and mechanisms for medical self-regulation.

> ... British clinical skills have been well-regarded internationally and since the mid 1980s the National Health Service has had a cadre of health service managers. It is striking that service development is noticeably absent from the repertoire of skills and even the most prestigious teaching hospital, or concerned health authority, would be hard-pressed to identify individuals or groups with the skills and remit for institutional or health service development. (p.145)

Finally, what the 'needs of the NHS' are requires further clarification. The King's Fund response to the consultation paper argued it had not attempted to define this in a systematic way:

> Implicit in the paper is the disaggregated tradition of medical science and clinical practice which focuses on sharply defined problems within particular services or particular clinical conditions. As a consequence, it does not explicitly acknowledge issues which run right across the whole Service, or broad parts of it, nor

> those which span the Service and other fields of public policy.[16]

A more general problem is that SDO-type research essentially deals with the behaviour of human beings in social contexts – the classic social science focus. Unlike science, social science does not focus on the unconscious workings of chemical substances or biological processes. Human interaction involves inherent unpredictability – the subjects of research are themselves agents of choice – which makes all 'science' in this field problematic. Furthermore, ethical issues arise in terms of how research should be conducted (true also for much clinical work), but also in terms of the political values of the researchers that can subtly influence how research projects are chosen and how results are used. This leads us to our final set of concerns.

USING THE RESULTS

Health-related research generates a vast amount of what can loosely be called knowledge. It was recognised from the very start of the R&D programme that what was 'known' was not necessarily used in practice. Accordingly, a large amount of effort has been devoted to assessing the significance of the available evidence through systematic reviews and encouraging the application of research findings within the NHS itself.

But although these activities are clearly important, they are not enough. Within the NHS, as Peckham has argued, the response task has been grossly underestimated:

> [Research] needs to be amplified and complemented by an effective and coherent service development function. The challenge of absorbing and imaginatively exploiting technologies and of implementing

and refining new policies, constitutes a massive developmental task, yet there is no dedicated capacity within the National Health Service capable of tackling these questions efficiently and responsively. (p.144–5)

A further omission has been the impact of the results of research on society at large. As noted above, social science research is inherently uncertain. But, in fact, it can be argued that no science can hope to attain a 'final' resolution about how the world works. Problems of perception, induction, prediction and values pervade scientific method in all its manifestations, and should lead us to be wary about proclaiming scientific knowledge as objective and uncontentious.[17] We cannot do justice to these themes in this article, but a number of current or recent examples – such as the BSE crisis, and fears over the safety of mobile phones, GM crops and stem cell research – indicate how science and scientists can simply get things wrong, or at least display very serious uncertainties about what is 'right'.

This is more than simply a matter of methodology. The examples given above are of profound interest to the general public. The recent case of fears over the safety of the MMR vaccine led to public concern and a consequent reduction in take-up, even when the overwhelming majority of scientists argued that the vaccine was safe, at least according to the best current evidence. It seems that the public has grown increasingly aware in practical terms of the underlying philosophical uncertainty of science. Examples of 'failures' emerge more clearly as public accountability, information technology, media interest and levels of education open up the previously closed worlds of all kinds of expert. This is inevitable in modern democracies, and most would argue a good thing too. But it may also reveal a disjunction between attitudes to societal change and risk of the general public and those of the professional researcher.

A recent report from the House of Lords Select Committee on Science and Technology[18] put it this way in its introduction:

> Society's relationship with science is in a critical phase. Science today is exciting, and full of opportunities. Yet public confidence in scientific advice to Government has been rocked by BSE; and many people are uneasy about the rapid advance of areas such as biotechnology and IT – even though for everyday purposes they take science and technology for granted. This crisis of confidence is of great importance both to British society and to British science.

Table 5: Public attitudes to science

Subject	per cent agreeing	
	2000	1996
Science and technology are making our lives healthier, easier and more comfortable	67	73
It is important to know about science in my daily life	59	51
Science makes our lives change too fast	44	53
The benefits of science are greater than the harmful effects	43	45

There is some survey evidence to support these contentions.[19]

In only one of these subject areas does confidence seem to have improved, with fewer people now agreeing that science makes lives change too fast. In all the other areas, the trend can be interpreted as one of weakening confidence. And, simply looking at the percentages in their own terms, it is perhaps surprising that less than half of those polled believe that science's benefits outweigh its costs.

In short, the average citizen's attitude to risk, to the appropriate focus of scientific advance and to the balance of benefits to potential costs, may well differ sharply from that of the scientific community and policy-makers. And this may not simply be a matter of misunderstanding but one of values and of interests – after all, the individual citizen does not stand to gain a Nobel Prize from the development of cloning technology. As a result, in a more open and democratic society we must now tackle the issue of how to manage the consumption of knowledge by the *whole* of society. Perhaps too little effort is devoted to thinking about how we cope with knowledge, and too much with simply going ahead and producing it.

To some extent these issues have been recognised. *The NHS Plan*[20] notes that:

> We now have the first provisional map of the human genome and innovation will occur at an ever faster rate. It is vital that the NHS plays an active and collaborative role in realising the benefits in genetics. We will contribute with other government departments and medical charities to a long-term study of the interactions of genetics and the environment in common diseases of adults such as cancer, heart disease and diabetes. These powerful techniques for

understanding and treating disease also raise important issues for society in general. The Government has already set up the Human Genetics Commission to advise on the social, ethical and legal implications of developments in genetics and to engage the public in considering these questions. (para. 11.14)

The point it makes, however, is of much more general application.

PART 4: CONCLUSIONS

The process for reforming the finance and management of the NHS R&D programme is still under way and some key elements have yet to appear. But it seems clear that, despite the vast effort that has been devoted to improving the way resources are used within it since 1988, a number of important issues continue to be systematically ignored.

The papers we have drawn on touch on most of them, but none receive systematic discussion or analysis. As a result, while the machinery for the finance of health-related research may be better, whether the programme as a whole can be justified remains uncertain.

In particular:

- Although much of the groundwork is in the process of being laid, there remains a lot to do before there can be confidence that the R&D funded from public sources represents the best attainable 'mix'.
- Similarly, the yet more complicated task of ensuring that the National Health Service as a whole obtains the best mix has yet to be thoroughly addressed.
- There should be more effort devoted to communicating and gaining

BOX 2: THE FINANCE OF CANCER RESEARCH

In 2000, the House of Commons Science and Technology Committee published *Cancer Research: a fresh look*. This report, the Government's response to it and the *Cancer Plan* published in September 2000 shed a great deal of light on the issues considered in this paper.

The Committee received evidence which suggested that the organisation of cancer research taken as a whole was poor, despite the excellence of some of its parts. It found that, despite the importance attached to cancer in *Research for Health*, the publicly-financed contribution to cancer care was less than that of other main funders.

It took the view that:

> Most UK cancer researchers receive far more support from the research charities and the pharmaceutical industry than they do from the Government. We believe that this imbalance is unhealthy. Notwithstanding the Government's wish to partner and co-operate with cancer research charities, if it does not fund research then the research which it wishes to see will not be done. Cancer research charities cannot and should not be expected to fund research as part of a national strategy. The Government has abdicated its responsibility for cancer research and has by default placed the research agenda in the hands of charities and industry. (para. 145)

It did not in fact believe the Government's own figures on cancer research funding:

> The conviction of many witnesses and of those we met on visits is that most of the NHS R&D funding was disappearing into general support for NHS hospitals and that little of it was actually made available for research purposes. This means that of the £112 million that the Government claims to spend on cancer research, more than half is effectively unaccounted for and may not be spent on research at all. This situation is deeply unsatisfactory. (para. 140)

In the light of the above it recommended an immediate increase of £100 million.

It also found that:

> There is widespread agreement that the poor state of the infrastructure for cancer treatment and research in the NHS is a serious barrier to clinical research. The Government must act quickly to address this through investment in the necessary staff, training, equipment and buildings. (para. 91)

It concluded that:

> If the pharmaceutical industry is to be encouraged to do more cancer clinical trials in this country the costs of doing so must be made competitive with those in other countries. (para. 129)

However, other evidence submitted to the Committee, e.g. from the Royal Pharmaceutical Society, suggested that research was being subsidised as vital support services were not usually covered in contracts.

democratic legitimacy for scientific developments, and honesty about the inherent uncertainties.

● Finally, although we cannot attempt in this paper to assess in detail how effective the new arrangements have been at redirecting R&D funds, two points can be made. First, the attempt to reduce the dominance of clinical research has yet to be effective: the SDO programme has scarcely got off the ground. Second, there has been little progress towards refocusing the R&D funds supported by the levy and paid direct to providers.

REFERENCES

1. House of Lords Select Committee on Science and Technology. *Medical Research and the NHS Reforms.* HL Paper 12, Session 1994–95, 3rd Report. London: HMSO, 1995.

2. From the DoH website www.doh.gov.uk/ research, 26 July 2000.

3. From www.doh.gov.uk/research/nrr.htm

4. House of Lords Select Committee on Science and Technology. *Priorities in Medical Research: Volume 1 – Report.* London: HMSO, 1988.

5. Department of Health. *Research for Health: A Research and Development Strategy for the NHS.* London: HMSO, 1991.

6. Department of Health Research and Development Task Force. *Supporting Research and Development in the NHS: a report to the Minister of Health.* A J Culyer (chair). London: HMSO, 1994.

7. Department of Health Central Research and Development. *Strategic Review of the NHS R&D Levy: Final Report.* London: Department of Health, 1999.

8. Department of Health. *NHS Priorities and Needs R&D Funding. A position paper.* London: HMSO, 2000.

9. Black N. A National Strategy for Research and Development: Lessons from England. *Annual Review of Public Health* 1997; 18: 485–505.

10. House of Commons Science and Technology Committee. *Cancer Research – A Fresh Look: Volume 1: Sixth Report and Proceedings of the Committee.* London: HMSO, 2000.

11. Arnold E *et al. Implementing the Culyer reforms in North Thames: final report.* London: Department of Health, 1999.

12. Buxton M, Hanney S. *Assessing Payback from Department of Health Research and Development: Preliminary Report: Vol 1: The Main Report.* Uxbridge: Brunel University, 1994.

13. House of Lords Select Committee on Science and Technology. *Complementary and Alternative Medicine.* London: HMSO, 2000.

14. Harrison A, Dixon J. *The NHS: Facing the Future.* London: King's Fund, 2000.

15. Peckham Sir Michael, ed. *The scientific basis of health services.* London: BMJ Publishing, 1996.

16. *King's Fund Response to R&D consultation,* London: King's Fund, 2000.

17. Richards S. *Philosophy and Sociology of Science: an introduction.* Oxford: Basil Blackwell, 1987.

18. House of Lords Select Committee on Science and Technology. *Science and Society.* HL Paper 38. London: HMSO, 2000.

19. Office of Science and Technology and the Wellcome Trust. *Science and the Public: A review of science communication and public attitudes to science in Britain.* London: DTI and Wellcome Trust, 2000.

20. Department of Health. *The NHS Plan: a plan for investment, a plan for reform.* London: HMSO, 2000.

W(h)ither the national GP contract?

Richard Lewis and Stephen Gillam

The NHS Plan has proposed some important changes to the contractual arrangements that govern general practice.[1] The expansion of personal medical services (PMS) pilots, the decision to restructure the general medical services contract and the announcement that a new resource allocation mechanism will be developed for primary care, all suggest that that the relationship between the State and general practice is set to change. What are the prospects for the general practitioners' contract?

The importance of 'independent contractor status', together with the national negotiating machinery, has long been deeply embedded in the psyche of Britain's family doctors. The overwhelming majority of general practitioners consider themselves self-employed and this 'arm's-length' relationship with the NHS was enshrined in the settlement between the British Medical Association (BMA) and the Government in 1948.[2] However, general practitioners' support for the national contract and that symbol of independence, the infamous 'Red Book' (the Statement of Fees and Allowances) has steadily eroded. So too has the power of the medical profession collectively to impose terms upon the Government. Negotiations over the 1990 contract demonstrated clearly and painfully that the BMA had lost its ability to veto primary care policy. In future, ministers expected to exert greater control over the activity of the nation's doctors.[3] Over the last decade a growing number of young doctors have begun to contemplate a future as salaried practitioners[4] and the advantages of the existing contract have been increasingly contested.[5]

The first wave of PMS pilots took flight in 1998.[6] What distinguished these experiments was that both the service specification and budget were explicitly based on a contract agreed between the health authority (the contract 'principal') and the pilot (the contract 'agent'). Classical contracting theory implies that to make providers accountable for implementing their principal's policy objectives, the contractual system must be so constructed that the agents accept such contracts, that they implement the contract (payments being dependent on providing discrete specified benefits to the principal), and that these benefits help realise the principal's policy objectives.[7] Experience with the NHS internal market led economists to question how far contracts resembled principal–agent relationships on the classical model.[8] Relational theory holds that contracts achieve flexibility not by defining all contingencies beforehand but by agreeing to agree later about changes in circumstances and by constructing adaptable governance arrangements that allow the emergence of stronger working relationships.[9] Either way, local contracting should ensure primary care that better addresses local health needs.[10] Local negotiation should strengthen the principal–agent relationship and lead to services that are more closely attuned to the requirements of health authorities and Primary Care Trusts (PCTs, which will hold all new PMS contracts) as well as national policy objectives. Local contracts make possible the introduction of new indicators, incentives and penalties.

The Government has now nailed its colours to the PMS mast. Successful pilots will be made permanent and a majority of general practitioners are expected to transfer to PMS contracts over the next four years without any pre-piloting.[11] This appears, yet again, to be a case of health policy marching bravely in advance of available evidence. The national evaluation of first wave PMS pilots is not due for completion until next year and only interim findings or small-scale studies have been published to date.[12] So what does the early research evidence tell us so far about the impact of local contracting?

Analyses of PMS service agreements suggest that few first wave contracts took advantage of the potential opportunities made available to them. More than two-thirds of first wave pilot contracts left services broadly as they were under GMS and three-quarters offered 'block' payments that were not sensitive to the quality or quantity of services provided.[13] Few contracts specified clinical quality targets or activities such as the use of particular clinical guidelines. Even fewer attempted to define outcome measures and they were largely devoid of detail on how to achieve greater financial efficiency.[14] Local contracting for primary medical services is clearly immature.

A new 'National Contractual Framework' has been produced by the NHS Executive that is mandatory for all third wave PMS pilots.[15] Given the experience of first wave contracting, a degree of standardisation may be beneficial. It is nonetheless paradoxical that 'local contracting' should be accompanied by a raft of central guidance that constrains the very freedom of local action that is supposed to define PMS pilots.[16] PMS contracts are already being portrayed as a means through which the Government can enhance central control of general practitioners. This may serve to slow the take-up of pilots and will strain the already delicate relationships between PCTs and their professional constituents.

General practice is thus faced with two alternative contractual futures. Are these models compatible, or must they compete until only one survives? Their co-existence is problematic and may lead to perverse outcomes. For example, the introduction of new salaried doctors under PMS, funded through national growth monies, may well lead to a shift of workload away from the remaining GMS doctors as patients re-register. This could cause the GMS contract as a whole to undershoot its target level of remuneration. Ordinarily, the annual balancing mechanism would increase fees and allowances for the following year by way of compensation. In effect, GMS doctors may be paid more for less work.[17]

Ministers have stated that GMS will remain for doctors that want it.[18] However, the *NHS Plan* has now made clear that this commitment may not extend to single-handed practitioners, who may be forced into PMS contracts. What happens to single-handed doctors who do not meet the requirements of their contract has not yet been addressed. The commitment to GMS of other practices may diminish for other reasons. The ability of the existing payment mechanisms to adjust year-on-year for variation in GMS activity may be compromised with the growth of PMS. In any case, the proposal to incorporate GMS non-cash-limited expenditure into a single allocation mechanism appears, at the very least, to complicate current arrangements to reimburse fees and allowances through the national contract.

To state that the future of GMS is uncertain is not the same as saying that PMS contracts will prevail – at least, not in their original form. The future holds out the prospect of a convergence of these two contract options. The individuality of the pilot contracts in the first two waves of PMS is set to give way to much greater standardisation. *The NHS Plan* proposes that PMS and GMS will share the same core contract framework. In its original incarnation, PMS is dead – long live PMS. The likeliest result is a newly-configured 'national' contract that allows more local discretion at the margins. In all this there are big risks for government. The cost efficiency of the NHS is often attributed to strong general practice, one source of which is its comprehensive financing mechanism. Whatever its defects, the Red Book has proved adaptable in directing the development of general practice.[19] Will new systems prove as flexible or as inexpensive?

REFERENCES

1. Secretary of State for Health. *The NHS Plan: a plan for investment, a plan for reform.* Cm 4818–I. London: The Stationery Office, 2000.
2. Klein R. *The New Politics of the NHS.* 3rd ed. London: Longman, 1995.
3. Day P. The State, the NHS and General Practice. *Journal of Public Health Policy* 1992; 13 (2): 165–79.
4. Electoral Reform Ballot Services. *Your Choices for the future: a survey of GP opinion.* London: GMSC, 1992.
5. General Medical Services Committee. *Core services: taking the initiative.* London: GMSC, 1996.
6. NHS Executive. *A guide to Personal Medical Services Pilots under the NHS (Primary Care) Act 1997.* London: NHS Executive, 1997.
7. Harden I. *The contracting state.* Milton Keynes: OUP, 1995.
8. Propper C. Agency and incentives in the NHS internal market. *Social Science and Medicine* 1995; 40. 1683–90.
9. Campbell D. The relational constitution of discrete contracts. In: Campbell D, Vincent-Jones P, editors. *Contract and economic organisation.* Aldershot: Dartmouth, 1996.
10. Sheaff R, Lloyd-Kendall A. Principal-agent relationships in general practice: the first wave of English Personal Medical Services pilot contracts. *Journal of Health Services Research and Policy* 2000; 5 (3): 156–163.
11. Secretary of State for Health. *The NHS Plan: a plan for investment, a plan for reform.* Cm 4818–I. London: The Stationery Office, 2000.
12. Leese B, Gosden T, Riley A, Allen L, Campbell S. *Setting out: Piloting innovations in primary care. Report on behalf of PMS*

National Evaluation Team. Manchester: NPCRDC, 1999.

13. Sheaff R. Contracting for primary care. In: Lewis R, Gillam S, editors. *Transforming Primary Care – personal medical services in the new NHS.* London: King's Fund, 1999.

14. Lewis R, Gillam S, Gosden T, Sheaff R. Who contracts for primary care? *Journal of Public Health Medicine* 1999; 21 (4): 367–71.

15. NHS Executive. *A contractual framework for Personal Medical Services – Third Wave Pilots.* London: NHS Executive, 2000.

16. Department of Health. *Personal Medical Services pilots under the NHS (Primary Care) Act 1997 – A comprehensive guide.* 3rd ed. London: NHSE, 2000.

17. Lewis R, Gillam S. What seems to be the trouble? *Health Service Journal* 2000; 27 July: 28–30.

18. NHS Executive. *Primary Care Trusts: establishing better services.* London: NHS Executive, 1999.

19. De Maeseneer J, Hjortdahl P, Starfield B. Fix what's wrong, not what's right, with general practice in Britain. *BMJ* 2000; 320: 1616–67.

POLICY ANALYSIS

Should private medical insurance be subsidised?

Carl Emmerson, Christine Frayne and Alissa Goodman

INTRODUCTION

The private health care sector forms a relatively small part of the system of health care in this country, but its importance has grown in recent decades. Compared to the 3.6 million people covered by private medical insurance (PMI) in 1980, there are approximately 6.4 million people covered today, and private-sector health spending accounts for approximately 16 per cent of total health spending. This proportion remains small by international standards, and despite the significant increases in funding allocated to the NHS over the next five years, many commentators have predicted a further increasing role for the private sector as the NHS continues to grapple with ever-increasing demands.

An important question arising from this is whether there should be active encouragement for such growth in the private sector by government. Until recently, the UK tax system contained two subsidies to PMI. The first encouraged those over 60 to take out PMI

by providing income tax relief at the basic rate, and the second encouraged employers to provide PMI as a benefit-in-kind to employees, as no employers' National Insurance contributions were payable on this (as well as some other) benefits. Both of these reliefs have been abolished by the current government.

Here we examine the case for the subsidy of PMI. To do this, we first set the context by comparing public and private spending on health care in the UK and other European and G7 countries. We then set out how ownership of PMI has grown over the last four decades, and describe the characteristics of those who currently own PMI. We next consider whether the Government should encourage the take-up of PMI, by addressing firstly, whether there are considerations of equity and 'fairness' which would suggest that PMI should be subsidised. We then go on to consider whether any tax subsidy to PMI is likely to be self-financing. In part, this depends upon how responsive individuals are to changes in the price of PMI. We go on to examine this issue by considering the effect of the removal of tax relief on PMI to the over-60s announced in the July 1997 Budget. Using a 'difference of difference' approach we are able to estimate the number of people who gave up their insurance policies as a result of this reform, and consider whether the cost of any increase in demand for NHS services resulting from this decline in private coverage was likely to outweigh the estimated £135 million annual cost of the subsidy.

PUBLIC AND PRIVATE SPENDING ON HEALTH

The UK's health care sector, at 6.7 per cent of GDP, takes the smallest share of national income of all the G7 countries. This is shown in Figure 1, which sets out OECD estimates of the share of national income taken by public health spending and private health spending in 1998 for these countries. The US is the biggest health spender amongst this group, with almost 14 per cent of its GDP going to health care. Germany and France also have relatively large health care sectors,

Figure 1: Public and total health expenditure as a percentage of GDP in the G7 countries, 1998

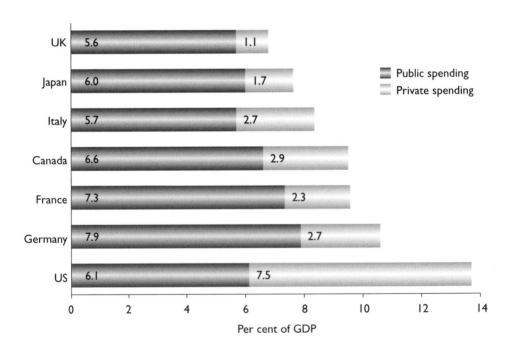

Note: Countries have been weighted by the size of their GDP. Currencies have been converted using 1998 exchange rates. An alternative methodology is to use purchasing power parities but in practice this makes little difference. For a discussion of the weighted and the less meaningful unweighted averages, see Chennells, Dilnot and Emmerson.[3]
Source: *OECD Health Data 2000: A Comparative Analysis of 29 Countries* (CD-ROM).

Table 1: Share of the private sector in total health care spending in the G7 countries, 1998

Country	Share of private sector (%)
US	55.3
Germany	25.4
France	23.6
Canada	30.4
Italy	32.0
Japan	21.7
UK	16.3

Note: Countries are ranked according to share of health spending in GDP.
Source: *OECD Health Data 2000: A Comparative Analysis of 29 Countries* (CD-ROM).

taking up 10.6 per cent and 9.6 per cent of their GDP respectively. Japan's and Italy's health care spending is closer to that of the UK, both with a public sector of similar size to ours but with a larger private sector in each case.

Partly as a response to the relatively low share of GDP spent on health care in the UK, the Government has pledged substantial real increases in NHS spending, averaging 6.2 per cent a year over the five-year period until March 2004. This is higher than the 3.4 per cent average real increase in spending that the NHS has received over its 50-year history.[1] The Prime Minister has also pledged that 'over time, we aim to bring it [NHS spending] up towards the EU average'.[2] Across the European Union average health spending in 1998 was 8.7 per cent of GDP, with the average (once the relatively low spending UK is excluded) being 9.1 per cent of GDP.[1] In fact, within the EU, only Luxembourg (5.9 per cent) and the Republic of Ireland (6.4 per cent) have a smaller health care sector than the UK. While the Government's planned increases in NHS spending could increase health spending

by 1.0 percentage point of GDP between 1998–99 and 2003–04, it is clear that these increases alone will not be sufficient to fully close the gap between UK health spending and the EU average by March 2004.

Another way in which the gap between health spending in the UK and that seen elsewhere could be closed is through growth in the role played by the private sector. Table 1 shows that while (from the point of view of spending) the private sector plays a role in the provision of health care in the UK, it is much smaller than the role played elsewhere. The US has by far the largest share of private spending amongst these countries, at 55.3 per cent. In Canada and Italy, the private sector accounts for around 30 per cent of health spending. In the UK, private spending amounts to just 16.3 per cent of the health sector, or roughly 1 per cent of our GDP.

The relatively small role played by the private sector in funding UK health care is largely due to the institutional set-up in the UK, where the publicly-funded NHS aims to provide free medical treatment through GPs and hospitals for all UK residents. In theory at least, any private spending on health is a matter of individual choice rather than need. For the substantial number of people who have private health insurance, combined use of private and public medical services is the norm. They are typically still reliant on the NHS for certain types of care, most notably for primary care and emergency care, which has stayed within the domain of the NHS. Use of private medical facilities is not restricted to those who are insured. An estimated 20 per cent of patients in the private sector pay for treatment themselves.[4] However, as we show in the following section, coverage of private medical insurance has grown substantially over the last 45 years and is now a prominent feature of the UK health system.

PRIVATE MEDICAL INSURANCE IN THE UK

Over the last 45 years, there has been a large increase in the number of people covered by PMI, as shown in Figure 1. In 1955, just over 0.5 million individuals were covered by PMI compared to a peak of 6.8 million in 1998. Two-thirds of the total increase in coverage since 1955 occurred between 1979 and 1990, since when it has remained roughly flat. Interestingly, between 1998 and 1999 coverage actually fell by 440,000, down to 6.4 million people, the largest fall in coverage of PMI seen in any one year since 1955.

Figure 2 also shows that two-thirds of PMI is actually provided through an employer rather than purchased directly by an individual. There are at least two

Figure 2: Number of people covered by private medical insurance, 1955–99

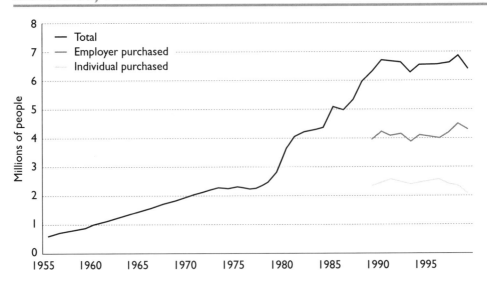

Notes: Data for whether the insurance was an employer or individual purchase are only available after 1989.

Sources: Office of Health Economics[5] for data prior to 1984; Laing and Buisson[6] for 1984 onwards.

reasons why it might be preferable to purchase health insurance through an employer rather than directly.

Firstly, a large employer is able to spread health risks across a large number of employees. This will help to mitigate the potential problem of adverse selection, where costs may escalate or the market may break down all together as only those individuals who are relatively likely to require health treatment decide to purchase insurance. This could potentially happen even if individuals did not know that they were more likely to be a bad health risk to the insurance company if, for example, they made their decision to purchase insurance after a parent or a sibling became ill.

Secondly, prior to April 2000, employers did not have to pay any employers' National Insurance on PMI. This gave employees an incentive to accept lower wages in return for insurance, rather than purchase it directly themselves.

CHARACTERISTICS OF THOSE WITH PRIVATE MEDICAL INSURANCE

Using data from the Family Resources Survey (FRS), we are able to construct a clearer picture of the individuals who have PMI.* Overall, 12.7 per cent of adults in the FRS are found to have PMI. This is similar to the 11.1 per cent of the population (i.e. including children) covered on average over the same five years in the published Laing and Buisson (L&B) data.[6] The FRS data also tells us whether the policy was paid for by

someone inside or someone outside the household, which we interpret as being paid for by an employer.** Unfortunately, the split between those reporting that they paid for the policy compared to those stating that someone else paid for the policy is not the same as in the industry L&B data. In the FRS data 57.8 per cent of individuals report that they paid for the policy, compared to one-third of those in the L&B data. This discrepancy could arise if some employers require a contribution from employees, or employers offer lower wages to employees who take up insurance, which is, unsurprisingly, interpreted by the individuals as them making a contribution rather than their employers.

Richer households are much more likely to have PMI than poorer households, as shown in Figure 3. Thus, 41.2 per cent of people in the richest 10 per cent of the population are privately insured, compared with under 3.7 per cent of those in the bottom 40 per cent. The likelihood of insurance being paid for by an employer increases with income. Thus, 50.7 per cent of those with health insurance in the top decile report that they have had it bought by an employer, compared with 25.5 per cent of those with health insurance in the bottom four income deciles. This is consistent with the idea that jobs which offer better remuneration are also more likely to offer other benefits, such as PMI. Another possible reason is that employers are more concerned about the health of more highly paid employees and hence are

---

*See Propper, Rees and Green[7] for a pseudo-cohort analysis of the demand for private medical insurance using the Family Expenditure Survey from 1978 to 1996. In addition, Propper[8] looks at actual use of private and public health care using the British Household Panel Survey. For more details of the FRS data see Appendix A.

** There may be situations where individuals are bought insurance by people, other than their employers, whom they do not live with (such as children or parents), although these cases are likely to be less important.

more likely to offer them packages that include PMI.

Coverage of PMI also varies by age and region, as shown in Table 2. The percentage of adults with insurance is lowest among the under-30s and the over-65s. Generational effects may be important too – evidence from Propper, Rees and Green[7] suggests that, while 30-year-olds are less likely to have PMI than 50-year-olds, 30-year-olds today are more likely to have it than 30-year-olds in the past. Table 2 also shows how coverage varies by region, with the proportions covered being highest in Greater London and the south-east, and lowest in the north.

In order to get a better understanding of the characteristics of those with and those without PMI, Table 3 presents some multivariate analysis. This shows that the age pattern observed in Table 2 still holds after the impact of other characteristics, such as income and employment status, is taken into account. We find that individuals in non-manual jobs are more likely to be insured independently of their income, although managers and technical staff are more likely to be insured than professionals. This is possibly due to the greater diversity of the 'professionals' group.

SHOULD THE GOVERNMENT ENCOURAGE THE TAKE-UP OF PRIVATE MEDICAL INSURANCE?

Increased use of private facilities can potentially ease the pressure on the NHS by freeing public spending that would otherwise have gone on those who have

Figure 3: Percentage of adults with private medical insurance, by income decile, 1995–96 to 1999–2000

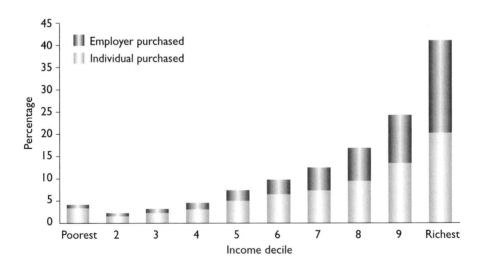

Sources: *Family Resources Survey*, 1995–96 to 1999–2000; authors' calculations.

Table 2: Percentage of people with private medical insurance, by age and region, 1995–96 to 1999–2000

	Age group					
Region	**< 30**	**30–39**	**40–49**	**50–64**	**65+**	**Total**
North	3.7	7.3	8.9	7.3	2.0	5.8
Yorks & Humberside	6.3	12.1	12.5	11.9	5.1	9.5
North-west	6.7	13.0	14.0	11.5	5.9	10.1
East Midlands	7.0	11.5	14.7	14.5	4.7	10.5
West Midlands	7.6	13.7	17.9	15.7	5.4	12.0
East Anglia	7.6	14.0	18.1	16.8	6.2	12.4
Greater London	13.8	20.8	20.8	18.9	9.9	16.9
South-east	13.1	24.1	27.4	26.2	13.1	21.0
South-west	6.8	12.0	15.5	16.3	9.2	12.1
Wales	4.7	9.4	11.4	10.0	4.0	7.8
Scotland	4.5	10.3	10.0	5.9	3.1	6.7
Total	8.5	15.4	17.2	15.7	7.2	12.7

Sources: *Family Resources Survey*, 1995–96 to 1999–2000; authors' calculations.

chosen to pay privately. In order to reduce demands on the NHS, the Government could encourage individuals to take out PMI, which would result in some treatment being paid for privately rather than through NHS spending. Previously, subsidies towards the cost of PMI have been implemented in two ways. First, prior to the July 1997 Budget, individuals aged over 60 received basic-rate tax relief on the purchase of PMI. This was regardless of whether they were actually income tax payers, and couples with one person aged 60 or over also qualified for the subsidy. Second, prior to April 2000, employers who purchased PMI for their employees did not have to pay any employers' National Insurance contributions on this benefit-in-kind.

The current Government has abolished all subsidies for those taking out PMI. The abolition of tax relief to the over-

60s, announced in the July 1997 Budget, raised an estimated £135 million in 1999–2000 for the Exchequer.[9] The measures announced in the March 1999 Budget, which removed the exemption from employers' National Insurance contributions on all benefits-in-kind that were already liable for income tax, raised a total of £415 million in 2000–01,[10] part of which is from the extension of employers NICs to employer-provided PMI.

The issue of whether to subsidise PMI can be considered from two points of view – first, by looking at what kinds of people gain from the removal of such subsidies and second, the effect these subsidies are likely to have on the NHS.

EQUITY CONSIDERATIONS

It can be seen as fair that those individuals who have chosen to pay for

Table 3: Characteristics of those with private medical insurance

Characteristic	Impact on likelihood of having private medical insurance
Age	Individuals aged between 40 and 65 are found to be the most likely to be covered by PMI, with those aged over 70 and under 30 being the least likely.
Family situation	Individuals living in households without children are more likely to be covered.
	Individuals living in households containing either adult children or unrelated individuals are 1.4 percentage points less likely to be covered by PMI than others.
Gender	Men are found to be more likely to be insured than women, by 1.0 percentage point.
Income	For the vast majority of the population, income has a positive effect on possession of PMI, but this effect is found to decrease at higher income levels.
Employment status	Employees are found to be more likely to have PMI than either the self-employed or those out of work.
Education	Compared with those who left education at the minimum school-leaving age, those with college education are more likely to have insurance, while those with just A-levels are even more likely to be covered. The group with the highest probability of being covered by insurance is those still in education. They are likely to be covered by their parents' policies.
Housing tenure	Individuals in owner-occupied accommodation are 5.3 percentage points more likely to have PMI than others.
Regions	Individuals in the West Midlands, Greater London and the south-east are most likely to have PMI.
Occupation	Those in non-manual jobs are most likely to possess medical insurance. Managerial and technical staff are the most likely to have medical insurance, followed by professionals and skilled non-manual workers. Those in the armed forces are the least likely.
Savings	Individuals with higher levels of savings are found to be more likely to be covered by PMI.

Notes: All these results are significant at the 95 per cent confidence interval. For more details, see Appendix A.

Sources: *Family Resources Survey*, 1995–96 to 1999–2000; authors' calculations.

PMI and hence 'opt out' of some parts of NHS cover should receive a tax refund. This subsidy could reflect the saving to the Government from an individual choosing to 'opt out' of the parts of the NHS covered by PMI packages. This would be similar in practice to the reduced rate of National Insurance contributions paid by individuals who have chosen to 'opt out' of the State Earnings Related Pension Scheme into their own private pension. There are, however, some complicated issues here, such as the extent to which PMI companies offer benefits over and above those offered by the NHS – for example private rooms and better choice of food. In addition, some PMI schemes overlap with State coverage – for example some only offer payments for conditions where waiting lists are above certain levels. Other schemes offer financial payment for insured individuals to take NHS treatment. The distributional effect of any potential subsidy should also be considered. The previous section provided details of those individuals who are more likely to have PMI. Among other things this showed that individuals covered by PMI were much more likely to be found towards the top of the income distribution and hence any subsidy given to those with PMI is likely to be regressive as long as higher expenditure on PMI among richer households is not mitigated by premiums taking a smaller proportion of their incomes. Those who would gain from any subsidy also tend to have higher levels of savings and are more likely to be owner-occupiers.

There are also concerns about the effect this might have on public willingness to contribute to the NHS through taxation. Research shows that those with PMI are less likely to support increases on public health spending, even after their other characteristics are taken into account.[11] This finding suggests that continued growth in private sector health care would have implications for the level of support for an NHS that is provided

universally free at the point of use. It is of particular significance that those with medical insurance are likely to have higher incomes. These individuals may be more vocal in their opinions about the use of public funds and their concerns may be of particular importance as they will be paying more tax than average. It should be noted, though, that support for the NHS within this group, while reduced, still remains high.

COULD A SUBSIDY TO PMI BE SELF-FINANCING?

The removal of these subsidies is likely to have led to a reduction in the numbers covered by insurance and hence an increase in demands on the NHS. For example, the price of PMI for those aged over 60 will have increased by 29.9 per cent as a result of the removal of the income tax subsidy.* Depending on how responsive the demand for PMI is to changes in its price – known as the price elasticity of demand – this will have led to a reduction in coverage of PMI and potentially an increase in demands on the NHS. It is also true that the money saved from the subsidy could, alternatively, have been spent directly on the NHS. An interesting question, therefore, is whether a subsidy to the purchase of PMI can ever be self-financing in the sense that its cost is outweighed by the savings made by the reduction in demands on the NHS.

A simple model can be used to show whether it is likely that any subsidy to the NHS is self-financing. The cost to the Government from subsidising PMI depends on the rate at which the subsidy is given (t), the average cost of buying PMI before the subsidy (P_1), the number of people who already take out PMI (N_1)

---

* The basic rate of income tax when relief was abolished in 1997 was 23 per cent, as opposed to the current level of 22 per cent, which was introduced in April 2000. This leads to a price increase 0.23/ (1–0.23), i.e. 29.9 per cent.

and the number of additional people who take out PMI as a result of the subsidy being offered (N_2). Hence, assuming that the subsidy does not affect the gross price of PMI,* then:

Cost of subsidy = $t \times P_1 \times (N_1 + N_2)$ (1)

The additional saving to the NHS will depend on the number of additional people who take out PMI as a result of the subsidy (N_2) and the average saving to the NHS from each of these individuals. This can be expressed as a proportion of the cost of these individuals purchasing PMI ($p - P_1$). The relative cost of the treatment these people will require if it is provided by the NHS compared with the cost of them purchasing PMI is represented by p.

Saving to the NHS = $p \times P_1 \times N_2$ (2)

It seems reasonable to assume that $0 \leq p \leq 1$. This is because $p = 0$ implies that there is absolutely no saving to the NHS from individuals who have taken out PMI. Values of p greater than 1 are only plausible if the PMI industry was able to provide health care more cheaply than the NHS. There are at least two reasons why p can be expected to be less than 1:

- **Quality of health care provided.** Individuals who have PMI will presumably expect to receive better quality, but more expensive, health care than that provided by the NHS. For example, in addition to patients not having to wait for treatment, PMI providers often point to other benefits – such as individuals being able to get additional facilities such as private rooms, en-suite bathrooms, televisions and telephones. To the extent to which these types of fringe benefits are not available on the NHS this will tend to reduce the saving to the NHS from each £1 of insurance bought.

- **Cost of providing health care.** Given the market power that the NHS is able to exert when setting the wages of doctors and nurses, it is likely that it will be able to deliver health care extremely cheaply. In 1993–94 the average hourly private sector wage across a range of specialties was at least three times higher than that in the NHS.[12] While the private sector may be able to deliver some aspects of health care more efficiently than the NHS,** it seems unlikely that the overall costs of each treatment will be lower.

There is evidence that equivalent treatment is more costly when undertaken by the private sector.[13] For example, a cataract extraction and lens prosthesis costs £1950 to £2600 when undertaken in the private sector compared with the NHS cost of £847, and a hip replacement costs £5800 to £7500 in the private sector compared with the NHS cost of £3678. This difference in price is due to both the quality and the costs of private sector care being higher than the NHS. This points towards the value of p being lower that 1, at least on the two procedures listed above.

---

* This depends on how important fixed costs are in the provision of both PMI and NHS care.
** Recent years have seen efforts to improve the internal efficiency of the NHS, for example through the introduction of the 'internal market' at the start of the last decade. Evidence on the effect of this reform is mixed,[14,15] but the purchaser–provider split is generally judged to have been a success and is being maintained, despite the abolition of the internal market, in the recent restructuring that has seen the creation of new Primary Care Groups.[16]

Evidence on the actual value of p is provided by Department of Health,[2] which estimates that 'for a 65-year-old, private health insurance costs around 50 per cent more than equivalent NHS cost'. This would imply a value of p of 0.67.[*]

Hence, for any subsidy given to PMI to be self-financing the cost (given in (1)) needs to be less than or equal to the saving (given in (2)):

$$t \times P_1 \times (N_1 + N_2) \leq P_1 \times N_2 \times p \qquad (3)$$

Re-arranging (3) implies that:

$$N_2 \geq t \times N_1 / (p - t) \qquad (4)$$

If a subsidy were given equal to the current basic rate of income tax and this is available to all individuals (i.e. t = 0.22), and given that, according to the latest Laing and Buisson data (*see Figure 2*) there are currently 6.37 million policyholders (i.e. N_1 = 6.37 million), then equation (4) implies:

$$N_2 \geq 0.22 \times 6.37 / (p - 0.22) \qquad (5)$$

If we take the more extreme assumption that p = 1, *for the subsidy to be self-financing this would need an additional* **1.8 million** *people to take out policies*. This is equal to growth in the market of 28 per cent. Smaller values of p would require even *more* individuals to take out insurance for the subsidy to be self-financing. For example, if the 0.67 value implied by the Department of Health[2] estimate was correct for the entire population, then for a 22 per cent subsidy to be self-financing would require PMI market growth of 49 per cent.[**] *This is*

equivalent to an additional **3.1 million** *subscribers.*

We can also work out the minimum required price elasticity for the subsidy to be self-financing.[***]

Again taking the more extreme assumption of p = 1, this requires the elasticity to be at least −1.28. Smaller values of p would require demand to be even more responsive to changes in price. Although there is little UK evidence on price elasticities for PMI, this required elasticity can be compared to known price elasticities, for example the price elasticity of beer (a relatively inelastic good) has been estimated at −0.76, whilst the price elasticity for wine (a more price-elastic good) has been estimated at −1.69.[17] The minimum price elasticity for PMI for the subsidy to be self-financing lies between these two. We can also obtain further information about the price elasticity of PMI by analysing the impact of the removal of tax relief on PMI for the over-60s in the July 1997 Budget. We turn to this next.

WHAT EFFECT DID THE ABOLITION OF A PMI SUBSIDY HAVE?

In the 1997 Budget, the Labour Government abolished tax relief on private medical insurance that had been previously offered to those aged 60 or over. The Government estimated that 550,000 people would be affected by this measure, raising a total of £135 million for the Treasury by 1999–2000.[****] The immediate effect of the abolition of tax relief was to increase the cost of PMI for

---

[*] Since $C / (1.5 \times C) = 0.67$.

[**] i.e. $0.22 / (0.67 - 0.22) = 0.49$.

[***] Elasticity $= \dfrac{-(P_1 / N_1) \times (t \times N_1 / [p - t])}{(t \times P_1)} = \dfrac{-1}{(p - 0.22)}$

[****] While one-third of a million policyholders lost tax-relief[9] these policies covered a total of 550,000 people. See Inland Revenue Press Release, *Tax relief for Private Medical Insurance to be ended*, 2 July 1997.

Table 4: Coverage of PMI among those receiving and those not receiving a subsidy

	Pre-reform	Post-reform	Difference
Aged under 60	13.8	14.6	0.8
	(0.1)	(0.2)	(0.2)
Aged 60 or over	9.2	8.8	−0.4
	(0.2)	(0.2)	(0.3)
Difference	4.6	5.9	
	(0.2)	(0.3)	
Difference in difference estimate			−1.2
			(0.4)

Note: Standard errors contained in parentheses.
Sources: *Family Resources Survey*, 1995–96 to 1999–2000; authors' calculations.

all over-60s by 29.9 per cent of the price they were paying previously.* In Table 4 we show the percentage of people covered by PMI pre-reform and post-reform according to their age. We consider the pre-reform period to be prior to July 1997, when the policy was announced and introduced, while the post-reform period starts in July 1998. This one-year gap is due to the fact that many individuals have year-long policies, thus causing a lag between when the reform was introduced and when its full effect was felt.** Prior to July 1997, 9.2 per cent of those aged 60 or over*** were covered by PMI, while after July 1998 this number had fallen to 8.8 per cent of this age group.

Although there is no doubt that some of this decrease was due to the fact that

some individuals found the cost of PMI prohibitively high in the absence of the subsidy, other factors may also have affected people's decision as to whether to take out PMI. One such may have been whether there was any change in their expectation of the quality of care they would receive from the NHS in the short- and medium-term future. One way of looking at what would have happened to coverage of PMI had the subsidy not been abolished is to look at coverage among a group not affected by the reform. Prior to July 1997, 13.8 per cent of those under the age of 60 were covered by PMI, rising to 14.6 per cent after July 1998. In the absence of the reform we might therefore have expected the proportion of those covered aged 60 or over to increase by an equivalent amount – that is 0.8 percentage points – provided that trends

*The basic rate of income tax when relief was abolished in 1997 was 23 per cent, as opposed to the current level of 22 per cent, which was introduced in April 2000. This leads to a price increase of 0.23/ (1–0.23). Of course PMI prices may have been rising or falling over the period but 29.9 per cent represents the increase in price due to the removal of the subsidy.
** To qualify for the subsidy policies could not run longer than 12 months.
*** Or with a partner aged 60 or over.

in coverage occur similarly across both age groups. Using the under-60s to control for general trends in coverage of PMI suggests that the removal of the subsidy reduced the coverage among those aged 60 or over by 1.2 percentage points. Given that 550,000 people were covered by schemes prior to its abolition, this will have led to a reduction in coverage of 6600 individuals.

One problem with using the estimate calculated above is that it will be biased if the composition of the groups aged under 60 and 60 or over may have changed between the pre-reform and the post-reform period. Multivariate analysis allows us to look at the change in coverage between those aged 60 or over and those aged under 60 once other characteristics, such as income, educational attainment and housing tenure, are controlled for. This is the same technique used by Gruber and Poterba,[18] who evaluate the impact of the introduction of tax relief for the self-employed in the United States using employees as controls. Even if the characteristics of the under 60 and the 60 and over population have not changed, use of multivariate analysis may help to increase the precision of our estimates.

A probit model also allows us to get round the problem that we do not have information on the quantity of PMI that individuals have purchased. This is potentially important since some individuals may have introduced greater excess payments, or restricted the coverage of their insurance packages as a result of the removal of the government subsidy. The results of this are shown in Table A in Appendix A. We find that, once other observable characteristics are controlled for, the effect of abolishing the subsidy on PMI reduced the number of people covered by 0.7 percentage points amongst the eligible population. Given that 550,000 people were covered by schemes prior to its abolition, this will have led to a reduction in coverage of around 4000 individuals. The 95 per cent confidence interval is that coverage will have fallen by between 500 and 7200 individuals. *While this will have led to some increase in demands on the NHS, it is clear that this will be less costly than the £135 million saved by the abolition of the subsidy.*

The estimate of the price elasticity of PMI from our probit model is that a 29.9 percentage point increase in price led to a 0.7 percentage point fall in quantity demanded.* Hence the estimated price elasticity of PMI is –0.024, with a standard error of 0.01.** This gives a 95 per cent confidence interval of –0.003 to –0.044. This suggests that PMI is an extremely price inelastic good (i.e. changes in price having very little effect on demand). Furthermore, this estimated elasticity is substantially lower than the lowest required price elasticity of –1.28 to make PMI tax subsidy to be self-financing.

CONCLUSION

The last 20 years have first seen a ten-year period of extremely large growth in the numbers covered by PMI (from 3.6 million in 1980 to 6.7 million in 1990),

---

* The elasticity found assumes that prices will have been unchanged in the absence of the removal of the subsidy. In practice, PMI prices have in recent years tended to rise by more than inflation. Given that PMI coverage is below 50 per cent, the probit model implies that our estimate will tend to be an over-estimate of the responsiveness of demand for PMI to changes in price.
** The standard error of the elasticity is equal to $\sqrt{(((1-0.23)/0.23)^2 * 0.01^2)}$.

followed by ten years in which coverage has essentially remained flat. The rate of coverage is correlated with a variety of socio-economic characteristics, with those between the ages of 40 and 49 and higher-income individuals being more likely to possess insurance. For example, over 40 per cent of people in the top income decile are covered by PMI compared with under 5 per cent in the bottom four deciles. Moreover, the higher up the income distribution a person is, the more likely it is that their insurance has been provided by their employer.

The causes and implications of the trends in the coverage of PMI are both interesting and important from a public policy perspective. When considering why individuals might choose to buy health insurance, we obviously need to consider the link between the level and quality of NHS health care and the number of people purchasing PMI. For example, Calnan, Cant and Gabe[19] find that those with PMI are more likely to be dissatisfied with the NHS than those without it. Whether this is purely a cause or also partly an effect of those individuals being in possession of PMI is unclear. While it seems obvious that those who are dissatisfied with the quality of NHS provision will be more likely to purchase PMI, it is also highly plausible that some individuals may change their valuation of NHS provision after using private care paid for through employer-provided PMI.

One measure of the quality of NHS provision that does seem to be positively correlated with the greater purchasing of private health insurance is the length of waiting lists for NHS treatment. This could be an indication that waiting lists are a particular concern or, alternatively, that they are used as a barometer for NHS

performance.[20,21] The fact that there is a link between waiting lists and the purchase of PMI is perhaps not surprising, given the degree to which the media and political parties have focused on them.

Despite the increase in use of the private sector, private spending on health care makes up only 16.3 per cent of total health spending in the UK, which is lower than in any other G7 country. In 1998, UK health spending was 6.7 per cent of GDP, which is some 2.4 percentage points lower than the average of the other 14 EU countries. The Government is eager to redress this balance and large increases in NHS spending have been planned until March 2004. The result will be that NHS spending will increase by 1.0 percentage point of GDP between 1998–99 and 2003–04. While substantial, these increases alone will be insufficient to fully close the gap between the UK and the rest of the EU by March 2004. Another way of increasing total spending on health would be to encourage people to take out PMI. This would have the added effect of reducing the demands on the NHS. Some individuals with PMI would in effect 'opt out' of the NHS for the treatments they were covered for.

One possibility would be for the Government to encourage individuals to take out PMI by offering a subsidy. We have considered whether the introduction of such a rebate could actually be self-financing, in other words, whether the saving to the NHS could be greater than the level of subsidies paid by the Treasury. Our analysis shows that this is unlikely to be the case, largely because a subsidy would benefit current holders of PMI while the saving to the NHS would only stem from the additional policies that would be sold due to the subsidy. It is also the case that the purchase of PMI will lead to a decrease in demands on the NHS by less than the policy cost, as private health care is more costly due to the higher quality of care provided, for example through less waiting and greater provision of private rooms, and the higher costs faced by the private sector. Prior to 1997, such a subsidy existed for the over-60s – individuals with PMI received a subsidy equal to the basic rate of income tax on the cost of their insurance. We analyse the effect of the abolition of this subsidy on the demand for PMI and find that, on our best estimate, there was a 0.7 percentage point decrease in the number of people covered by such insurance. This is equivalent to nearly 4000 individuals. While this would clearly have led to increased demands on the NHS, the cost of treating these individuals is likely to have been substantially lower than the £135 million annual cost of the subsidy.

ACKNOWLEDGEMENTS

This research is funded by the Economic and Social Research Council as part of the research programme of the ESRC Centre for the Microeconomic Analysis of Fiscal Policy at IFS. The authors would like to thank Ian Crawford for helpful comments. Data from the Family Resources Survey were kindly supplied by the Department of Social Security. Responsibility for the interpretation of data, and any subsequent errors, is the authors' alone.

APPENDIX A: MULTIVARIATE ANALYSIS OF THE CHARACTERISTICS OF THOSE WITH PRIVATE MEDICAL INSURANCE USING THE FAMILY RESOURCES SURVEY

The Family Resources Survey (FRS) is an annual survey of around 45,000 individuals that combines information on basic characteristics, such as family structure and employment status, with detailed income information. Although it does not contain information on direct expenditure on private medical treatment, the FRS records whether individuals are covered by PMI. We use combined FRS data for 1995–96 to 1999–2000 covering 214,334 individuals. Table A gives the results of multivariate analyses on the characteristics of those with PMI.

Table A: Individuals with private medical insurance

Characteristic	Probability of having private medical insurance	
	Coefficient	t-statistic
Interviewed between July 97 and July 98	0.003	1.05
Interviewed after July 97	−0.002	0.93
Aged 60 or over[a]	0.000	0.00
Interviewed between July 97 & July 98 & aged 60+[a]	−0.003	0.74
Interviewed after July 97 and aged 60+[a]	−0.007	2.20
Age	−0.017	5.08
Age ^{2} – squared	0.001	5.35
Age ^{3} – cubed	−0.000	5.10
Age ^{4} – power 4	0.000	4.51
Partner's age	0.018	3.34
Partner's age ^{2} – squared	−0.000	2.80
Partner's age ^{3} – cubed	0.000	2.32
Partner's age ^{4} – power 4	−0.000	1.95
Living with a partner	−0.293	3.52
Male	0.010	7.36
Other adult in household	−0.014	8.84
Person has child	0.021	11.61
Income / 1000	0.317	67.06
(Income / 1000) squared	−0.085	40.20
(Income / 1000) cubed	0.006	27.87
Employee	0.032	15.60
Self-employed	0.007	1.77
Owns home	0.053	32.15
Educated to A-level	0.038	21.42
College-educated	0.032	16.58
Still in education	0.107	13.31
Other information included	Chi–squared	p-value
Occupational dummies	768.94	0.000
Regional dummies[b]	1914.48	0.000
Household savings	357.61	0.000
Interaction of savings with having a partner	49.98	0.000
Year dummies	12.11	0.007
Month dummies	26.33	0.006
No. of observations	214,334	
Pseudo R-squared	0.197	

Note: [a]Or has a partner aged 60 or over. [b]Greater London and the south-east being the areas with the highest rates of coverage. A full set of results is available from the authors upon request.

REFERENCES

1. Emmerson C, Frayne C, Goodman A. *Pressures in UK Health care: Challenges for the NHS*. Commentary no. 81. London: Institute for Fiscal Studies and King's Fund, 2000.

2. Department of Health. *The NHS Plan: a plan for investment, a plan for reform*. Cm 4818-I. London: The Stationery Office, 2000.

3. Chennells L, Dilnot A, Emmerson C. *IFS Green Budget: January 2000*. Commentary no. 80. London: Institute for Fiscal Studies, 2000.

4. Office of Fair Trading. *Health Insurance*. London: OFT, 1996.

5. Office of Health Economics. *Compendium of Health Statistics*. 11th ed. London: OHE, 1999.

6. Laing and Buisson. *UK Market Sector Report 2000*. London: Laing and Buisson Publications Ltd, 2000.

7. Propper C, Rees H, Green K. *The demand for private medical insurance in the UK: a cohort analysis*. Working Paper no. 99/013. Bristol: University of Bristol, Centre for Market and Public Organisation, 1999.

8. Propper C. *The demand for private health care in the UK*. mimeo. Bristol: University of Bristol, Department of Economics, 1999.

9. HM Treasury. *Equipping Britain for our long-term future: Financial Statement and Budget Report, July 1997*. Hc85. London: HM Treasury, 1997.

10. HM Treasury. *Building a Stronger Economic Future for Britain: Financial Statement and Budget Report, March 1999*. Hc298. London: HM Treasury, 1999.

11. Brook L, Hall J, Preston I. What drives support for higher public spending? In: Taylor-Gooby P, editor. *Choice and Public Policy: The Limits to Welfare Markets*. London: MacMillan, 1998.

12. Monopolies and Mergers Commission. *Private Medical Services*. Cm 2452. London: HMSO, 1994.

13. Hennell T. People covered by private health insurance will not reduce consumption of NHS services. Letter. *BMJ* 2000; 321 (7265): 898.

14. Le Grand J, Mays N, Mulligan J. *Learning from the NHS Internal Market: A Review of the Evidence*. London: King's Fund, 1998.

15. Propper C, Croxson B, Perkins A. Do doctors respond to financial incentives? UK family doctors and the GP fundholder scheme. *Journal of Public Economics* 2001; 79 (2): 375–98.

16. Department of Health. *The New NHS: Modern, dependable*. Cm 3807. London: The Stationery Office, 1997.

17. Crawford I, Smith Z, Tanner S. Alcohol taxes, tax revenues, and the Single European Market. *Fiscal Studies* 1999; 20 (3): 287–304.

18. Gruber J, Poterba J. Tax incentives and the decision to purchase health insurance: evidence from the self-employed. *Quarterly Journal of Economics* 1994; 109 (3): 701–33.

19. Calnan M, Cant S, Gabe J. *Going Private: Why People Pay for their Health Care*. Oxford: Oxford University Press, 1996.

20. Besley T, Hall J, Preston I. *Private Health Insurance and the State of the NHS*. Commentary no. 52. London: Institute for Fiscal Studies, 1996.

21. Besley T, Hall J, Preston I. The demand for private health insurance: do waiting lists matter? *Journal of Public Economics* 1999; 72: 155–81.

Funding health care in Europe: recent experiences

Anna Dixon and Elias Mossialos

INTRODUCTION

Discussions about how to fund health care are not new in the UK. Indeed, the Government set up a committee of enquiry into the cost of the NHS as early as 1953. Chaired by C W Guillebaud, its terms of reference were to 'review the present and prospective cost of the National Health Service'. It concluded that if the NHS were to meet every demand that was justified on medical grounds it would require 'very considerable additional expenditure'.[1] Debates about changes to the system of funding the NHS also took place within the Conservative Government in the 1980s. A leaked paper prepared by the right-wing think-tank Centre for Policy Review Studies (CPRS), which proposed replacing the tax-financed NHS with a social insurance scheme, caused cabinet dissent and a public outcry, and led to the decision to concentrate on reforming the structure of the NHS rather than its financing.[2] More recent debates were precipitated by the 'winter crisis' in 1999–2000. The Labour Government has, however, reasserted its commitment to taxation in the NHS Plan.[3] In these debates about alternatives, such as social health insurance, or the role of private health insurance and user charges, examples from Europe are often cited.

However, many of these are based on anecdote or out-dated perceptions rather than facts.

In this article we review some of the recent and significant changes to health care funding in Europe. We analyse recent trends and draw some tentative conclusions about the significance of these for the debate in the UK.

HOW MUCH IS SPENT ON HEALTH CARE?

One of the main ways in which the UK is compared to other countries is on the basis of how much is spent on health. Despite the fact that such data are often presented as black-and-white facts, they are subject to a number of methodological and interpretative problems.[4] In brief, these include the definition of the boundaries of health care, the way definitions are standardised across countries, data collection methods, and differences in structure and organisation. There are also problems associated with the measurement and reporting of expenditure as a percentage of GDP. These estimates may vary, and no account is taken of the informal sector in the economy. Alternatives such as the use of exchange rate conversions and purchasing power parities (PPPs) when comparing per capita expenditure on health care have their own difficulties due to the basis of the calculation – the prices and basket of goods used are pharmaceutical-biased. Expenditure data should thus be interpreted with some caution.

Health care expenditure (HCE) as a percentage of GDP has stabilised in the latter part of the 1990s and even declined in some EU countries (see Table 1). However, in eight of the 15 EU countries GDP grew faster than HCE between 1995 and 1998, and in Spain, Portugal, Greece and Denmark HCE grew only a fraction more than GDP. Thus, the stabilisation of HCE as a percentage of GDP in some EU countries may not reflect success in controlling HCE growth but, rather, may be a reflection of growth in the economy. Indeed, in Ireland, while HCE grew by 3.4 per cent between 1995 and 1998, the economy grew by 8.8 per cent.[5]

Taking into account methodological limitations, the data show that the UK has consistently spent less in total than most other EU countries throughout the 1990s, ranking in the bottom three countries in any particular year. In terms of public expenditure on health, the UK consistently ranks in the lower half of countries. These data support the criticism that the UK health care system has suffered from chronic underfunding despite a period of economic growth. However, it is by no means certain that higher spending in some EU countries has resulted in more equitable or efficient systems.

WHERE DOES THE MONEY COME FROM?

Health care in Europe relies mainly on public funding; either from taxation or social health insurance. The third significant element is out-of-pocket expenditure. This includes both user charges paid in the public system and also direct payments for services provided in the private sector. The smallest proportion of private expenditure in nearly all countries (with the exception of the Netherlands) is private health insurance. Countries can be clustered into three groups according to the source of funding (see Figure 1): those that are predominantly funded through taxation (local taxes in Denmark and Sweden, central taxes in Italy,* Portugal, Spain, and the UK); those predominantly funded through social health insurance contributions (France,** Germany and the Netherlands); and those that are mixed systems (i.e. funded almost equally from tax and social health insurance) such as Belgium, Greece and Switzerland. It is worth noting that due to the organisation of the funding and pooling arrangements and historical origins, Belgium is often classified as a social health insurance system, Greece as tax-funded and Switzerland as privately-funded. Since 1996, Switzerland has moved away from voluntary private health insurance with individual risk-rated premia and variable packages of care, to a system of compulsory insurance provided by both private and public insurers with a guaranteed package of care and community-rated premia.

---

* Italy finances health through general and hypothecated tax, which is currently collected and set nationally. However, reforms are being introduced to decentralise the responsibility for health care funding to the regions.
** France is increasing the contribution of taxes to the funding of health care, as we discuss in more detail below.

Table 1: Total health care expenditure (public health care expenditure) as a percentage of GDP in EU member states, 1990–98

	1990	1991	1992	1993	1994	1995	1996	1997	1998
Austria	7.2 (5.3)	7.2 (5.3)	7.6 (5.6)	8.1 (6.0)	8.1 (6.0)	8.9 (6.4)	8.9 (6.3)	8.2 (5.8)	8.2 (5.8)
Belgium	7.4 (6.6)	7.8 (6.9)	7.9 (7.0)	8.1 (7.2)	7.9 (7.0)	8.2 (7.3)	8.6 (7.6)	8.6 (7.7)	8.8 (7.9)
Denmark	8.4 (7.0)	8.3 (6.9)	8.4 (7.0)	8.7 (7.2)	8.5 (6.9)	8.2 (6.8)	8.3 (6.8)	8.2 (6.8)	8.3 (6.8)
Finland	7.9 (6.4)	9.0 (7.3)	9.1 (7.3)	8.3 (6.3)	7.8 (5.9)	7.5 (5.7)	7.7 (5.8)	7.3 (5.5)	6.9 (5.3)
France	8.8 (6.7)	9.0 (-)	9.2 (-)	9.7 (-)	9.6 (-)	9.8 (7.5)	9.7 (7.4)	9.6 (7.3)	9.6 (7.3)
Germany	8.7 (6.7)	9.1 (7.1)	9.7 (7.6)	9.7 (7.5)	9.8 (7.6)	10.2 (8.0)	10.6 (8.3)	10.5 (8.0)	10.6 (7.9)
Greece	7.6 (4.8)	7.9 (4.8)	8.3 (4.9)	8.3 (4.8)	8.3 (4.9)	8.3 (4.8)	8.3 (4.9)	8.5 (4.9)	8.3 (4.7)
Ireland	7.0 (5.0)	7.4 (5.4)	7.8 (5.6)	7.8 (5.7)	7.7 (5.5)	7.4 (5.4)	7.2 (5.2)	7.0 (5.3)	6.4 (4.8)
Italy	8.1 (6.3)	8.4 (6.6)	8.5 (6.5)	8.6 (6.3)	8.4 (5.9)	8.0 (5.4)	8.1 (5.5)	8.4 (5.7)	8.4 (5.7)
Luxembourg	6.6 (6.1)	6.5 (6.0)	6.6 (6.1)	6.7 (6.2)	6.5 (6.0)	6.3 (5.8)	6.4 (5.9)	6.0 (5.5)	5.9 (5.4)
The Netherlands	8.8 (6.1)	9.0 (6.4)	9.2 (6.8)	9.4 (7.0)	9.2 (6.8)	8.9 (6.5)	8.8 (6.0)	8.6 (6.0)	8.6 (6.0)
Portugal	6.4 (4.2)	7.0 (4.4)	7.2 (4.3)	7.5 (4.7)	7.5 (4.8)	7.7 (5.0)	7.7 (5.1)	7.6 (5.1)	7.8 (5.2)
Spain	6.9 (5.4)	7.0 (5.5)	7.4 (5.8)	7.6 (6.0)	7.4 (5.9)	7.0 (5.5)	7.1 (5.5)	7.0 (5.4)	7.1 (5.4)
Sweden	8.8 (7.9)	8.7 (7.6)	8.8 (7.7)	8.9 (7.7)	8.6 (7.3)	8.4 (7.2)	8.7 (7.4)	8.5 (7.2)	8.4 (7.0)
UK	6.0 (5.1)	6.4 (5.4)	6.9 (5.9)	6.9 (6.0)	7.0 (5.9)	7.0 (5.9)	7.0 (5.9)	6.7 (5.6)	6.7 (5.6)

Source: OECD Health Data, 2000

Figure I

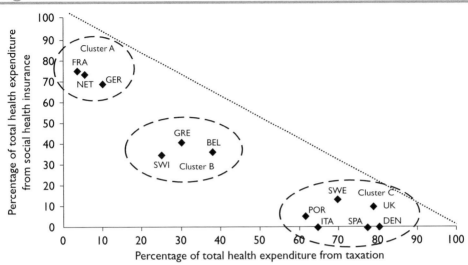

The pros and cons of each method of funding, for example the implications in terms of equity and efficiency, are discussed in detail elsewhere.[6–9] It is important, though, to note that even where a system is predominantly funded through taxation it may be regressive due to the significant use of user charges (e.g. Italy and Portugal).

Private expenditure accounts for as little as 11.4 per cent of total health expenditure (THE) in the UK but over 30 per cent of total health expenditure in Italy, Greece, Portugal and Switzerland. In all EU member states, except the Netherlands, the majority of private health expenditure is out-of-pocket payments and user charges. The smallest private health insurance markets are in southern Europe and Scandinavia. Private health insurance is also only a small percentage of total health expenditure in Belgium (2 per cent) and indeed in the UK (3.5 per cent). Private health insurance is more important in the Netherlands (17.7 per cent of THE), where it is the sole form of cover for those with incomes in excess of a defined ceiling, and in Germany (6.9 per cent of THE), where those with incomes above a defined ceiling are free to opt out of the statutory insurance scheme. In France, private health insurance accounts for 12.2 per cent of THE and is widely purchased to cover the co-payments within the public system. In Ireland (9.4 per cent) and Austria (7.1 per cent), private health insurance is purchased to cover additional services not available through public insurance for all the population. In several of these countries, not-for-profit as well as for-profit insurers are important. In France and the Netherlands not-for-profit insurers account for 64 per cent and 34 per cent of total private health insurance expenditure respectively.

The organisation of health care funding is not static; indeed, there have been a number of significant changes in recent years. These have not seen convergence between health care systems; indeed, both the objectives and direction of change vary. The main objectives that lie behind the funding reforms in Europe include a reduction in high labour market costs (e.g. France, Germany), a desire to promote choice and encourage competition in order to increase efficiency (e.g. the Netherlands), the provision of universal coverage for the population (e.g. France, Belgium and southern European countries), reduction of public spending either through the exclusion of services (e.g. over-the-counter drugs, dental care in most EU countries) or by increasing co-payments, and decentralisation of the funding of services (e.g. Italy). Here we highlight some of the most significant trends in both the method and organisation of health care funding in Europe:

- a shift from social health insurance to tax funding in France
- the introduction of insurer competition in Germany and the Netherlands
- the lack of significant growth in the private health insurance market in the 1990s
- increases in user charges and direct payments in several countries resulting from the (partial) exclusion of services from public cover.

SHIFT FROM SOCIAL HEALTH INSURANCE TO TAX FUNDING IN FRANCE

France has recently embarked on reform of health care funding. It is moving away from reliance on social insurance contributions towards a system funded through hypothecated taxes and from a system where eligibility was based on employment to one based on citizenship. The main justification for the diversification of funding sources was the potential negative impact of social insurance on industry. Social insurance contributions were believed to inhibit job creation (international comparisons have shown employment growth in France lagged behind other OECD countries). High wage costs were thought also to deter direct foreign investment.

The proposals, which were announced in November 1995 by the then Prime Minister Alain Juppé, formed part of a broader reform of the French social security system. Economic recession had left the social security budget in chronic deficit since 1991. The reform was therefore also driven by a desire to reduce the deficit and contain public expenditure. The main proposals in the areas of health care funding were as follows:

- reduction in the employee contribution from 5.5 per cent (1997) to 0.75 per cent of income (2000), combined with an increase in the general social contribution (GSC) tax (first introduced in 1991) from 3.4 per cent up to 7.5 per cent (depending on type of income) and earmarking this for health care
- introduction of a new social debt tax (*Remboursement de la Dette Sociale*) of 0.5 per cent on all income except social assistance and invalidity pensions
- parliament to be given the power to set a global budget for health care*

---

* This required a constitutional amendment and signified a major shift in power from the social partners who managed the social insurance system to the State.

- establishment of universal health insurance to extend the same benefits to all French residents over 18 years old.[10,11]

Known as the Juppé Plan, these proposals were developed secretly by four special advisers and high-level civil servants, the Prime Minister and the President of the Republic, thus by-passing the usual consultation with interest groups and stakeholders such as trades unions and professional groups. The reactions to the legislation were mixed. The main opposition to the reforms came from the trades unions: 'In general we oppose the tendency towards shifting financing from contribution to taxation. The transfer of financial obligations to the state will imply the transfer of decision-making power, and we are against that.'[12] Under the existing system, trades unions had majority representation on the boards of the funds and were in a powerful position vis-à-vis the government and employers. Under the Juppé Plan, membership of the boards would be split equally between the employers and the employees' representatives, namely the trades unions. There would also be a number of government-appointed members. With the change in funding, the link between employment and social benefits is broken and the role of the trades unions within the system less justified, while control by State and government is enhanced. The industrial action and public opposition to the social security reforms, of which the changes to health care funding were a part, led to the surprise defeat of Juppé at the next election. Radical change can have important political consequences.

Although the proposals were put forward by a centre-right prime minister, they elicited cross-party support as the principal ideas were social democratic in orientation and they were pursued by a new left-wing government elected in June 1996. The reforms have benefited from sustained cross-party support, as they are seen to be in the economic interests of the country and reduce the burden on labour. Following the introduction and expansion of the earmarked personal income tax, concern in France now centres around the equity implications of such heavy reliance on a proportional rather than a progressive income tax.

INSURER COMPETITION IN SOCIAL HEALTH INSURANCE SYSTEMS

In contrast to France, the Netherlands and Germany continue to rely predominantly on social health insurance. However, they have implemented significant changes to the organisation of social insurance. Up until the 1990s, in all western European countries with social health insurance systems there was more than one sickness fund but little choice, since people were assigned to funds on the basis of their geographical location, occupation or both. The latest trend, most notable in Germany and the Netherlands, has been to expand choice of funds.

In the Netherlands, the introduction of competition was part of an evolving debate on the role of competition that began as early as the 1940s. It mainly centred on concerns to increase the efficiency of the funds and it was expected to lead to rationalisation within the social health insurance system. The concrete proposals were put forward in the report of a government committee, chaired by W Dekker, former Chief Executive of Philips. The changes to the health insurance sector formed part of a wider restructuring of sick leave and disability insurance. Not all of the

Figure 2: Funding flows in the Dutch health care system

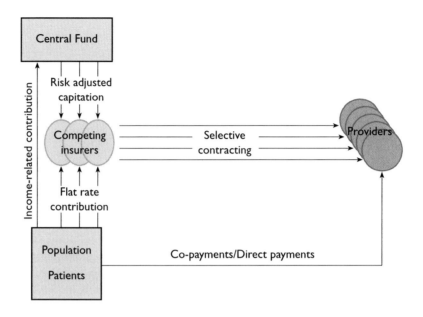

committee's recommendations were adopted, owing to doubts about the ability of the new system to contain costs and strong opposition from interest groups such as the private insurers and employers. However the following proposals were adopted:

- insurers were able to directly levy a flat-rate contribution set by them, in addition to the proportional income-based contribution, collected by the central fund, and the same for everyone regardless of insurer (Figure 2 illustrates how this operates)
- regional restrictions on sickness-fund activity (that had resulted in natural monopsonies) were abolished and new entrants, including private insurers, were allowed into the market

- insurers were allowed to contract selectively with providers and negotiate reimbursement prices lower than those set by the Central Tariff Authority (no insurers were able to do this due to the collusion and strength of the providers)
- insurers were able to restrict the purchase of supplementary insurance products to those subscribers who already had their main insurance from them.[13,14]

In practice, it is not clear from initial assessments to what extent insurer competition is having the desired impact. Because the value of the flat-rate contribution is relatively small (about NLG216, equivalent to £62 per year) and does not reflect the true costs of the insurance, price competition is very limited. It is likely that other factors such as a conveniently located insurance office or choice of fund of other family members will have more impact. The number of people who exercise their right to move funds is very small but has been increasing since the introduction of competition.[15]

One effect of the changes has been the emergence of private insurers who are active in the statutory insurance market. The established sickness funds, however, continue to dominate regional markets for statutory insurance. Choice of fund has prompted an accelerated process of mergers and acquisitions, and between 1985 and 1993 the number of insurers fell from 53 to 26. By 1999, there were 30 funds operating nationwide, with an average membership of about 300,000 persons (with a large variation in membership, ranging from less than 1000 to over 1 million). This suggested that when faced with competition, multiple insurers merged to benefit from economies of scale.[16]

Prior to 1996, German social health insurance was partly segmented according to occupation, and thus there were large differentials in contribution rates between the sickness funds (e.g. high-risk occupational groups were subject to the highest rates).* The Health Care Structure Act (GSG), which was passed in 1992 and came into effect in 1993, marked a major structural change in social health insurance. It granted equal legal status to manual and salaried workers (i.e. extended the right to change funds) and introduced cross-subsidisation between funds. In Germany, the

expansion of choice of sickness fund to all workers was partly motivated by a desire to reduce labour costs and to reduce the variation in contribution rates. However, the reform proposals also formed part of the political negotiations surrounding unification. Choice of fund for blue-collar workers was a prerequisite for the Social Democrats to accept the Solidarity Pact between West and East Germany.

The impact of the expansion of choice of fund in Germany was a reduction in variation in contribution rates. In 1994, 27 per cent of all members paid a contribution rate differing by more than 1 per cent from the average. This has reduced to only 7 per cent of all members in 1999 following enactment of the legislation. Data shows a shift away from the AOKs (general funds) (a net loss of 1.2 million members from 1997–99) to BKKs (occupational funds) (a net gain of 1.8 million members over the same period), which correlates with contribution rates.[17] Population surveys showed that in Spring 1999 only 7.3 per cent of the population had changed funds since 1996. Those who switched are more likely to have no dependants, to be from the former East Germany, under 40 years old and without chronic conditions. Price was mentioned most frequently by respondents as the reason for switching fund. Other reasons mentioned frequently were changing job, recommendation of a friend or acquaintance, unhappiness with the service and better coverage through the new fund.[18] However, it was not the explicit intention of the reform to encourage as many members as possible to change sickness funds but, on the contrary, that funds should be made to act

---

* In Germany, choice of funds already existed for white-collar workers but not for the majority of blue-collar workers.

more decisively in the interests of the insurees, above all by actively influencing the quality and efficiency of health care services. Their success in achieving this is more difficult to measure.

Multiple competing insurers may engender greater efficiency but may also bring potential difficulties in ensuring equal access to care for all. Therefore, in order to protect equity, insurers are required to accept all applicants. To stop some insurers from bearing a disproportionate part of the risk or adopting covert forms of cream-skimming, a mechanism for adjusting for risks is required. Risk adjustment in the Netherlands is performed by the central fund, which collects contributions from employers and employees. It then makes adjusted capitation payments to the funds. In Germany, where contributions are collected directly by the sickness funds, the adjustments are made by low-risk funds giving money to high-risk funds. Thus, the transfers are more visible in the German system.

PRIVATE HEALTH INSURANCE

The structure of private health insurance markets varies considerably between EU member states but growth in the private health insurance market has been stagnant in recent years. There are several reasons why this might be the case:

- the State continues to provide comprehensive benefits
- participation in the statutory health sector is compulsory in all countries (with some exemptions for some income/professional groups in Germany, the Netherlands and Spain)
- governments have tended to rely more on user charges as a method of shifting health care costs onto consumers,

rather than promoting and subsidising private health insurance
- consumers' preference to pay their doctor or hospital directly, rather than entrust a third party in southern Europe.[19]

Growth has mainly been in the group insurance sector, where premiums are usually cheaper (partly because of the greater purchasing power of an employer but also because risks are spread across all employees, i.e. there is group rating). There is no deliberate or explicit policy of encouraging individuals to take out private health insurance through the use of tax subsidies in seven of the EU member states. Voluntary health insurance receives generous tax relief in Ireland. Given at the standard rate of income tax (27 per cent), tax subsidies of VHI cost the Government £50 million a year (2.5 per cent of public expenditure on health in 1997). However, some countries have removed such incentives, especially for wealthy/high-rate taxpayers. Examples include Austria, where since 1996 private health insurance premiums are no longer tax deductible for those with annual incomes over SCH700,000 (equivalent to about £32,000), and in Spain where the 15 per cent tax deduction on premiums for medical expenses insurance was abolished in 1999.[19]

The role of the private health insurance market is more significant in Germany and the Netherlands, where it is the sole form of cover for a section of the population. This is not a recent change but has been the character of health insurance for a long time. In Germany, those who are eligible (i.e. with annual income over DM77,400 (£25,000) for those living in western Länder and DM63,900 (£21,000) for those in eastern

Länder) may choose to opt out of the statutory scheme and purchase private health insurance. In the Netherlands, all those people whose annual income exceeds NLG64,600 (around £19,000) are excluded from the statutory health insurance scheme. Nearly 98 per cent of them purchase private health insurance; the remainder choose to pay out of pocket.

The choice to remain in the statutory system or to purchase private health insurance is open for about 21 per cent of the German population (the self-employed are excluded from the statutory scheme, as are permanent public employees). In total, 7 per cent of the population (or 7.1 million people) choose full-cover private health insurance,* while 14 per cent of the population are voluntary members of the statutory scheme. In other words, only a third of those who are eligible to go private choose to do so. Private schemes are likely to be more attractive, particularly for single people or couples where both partners work. However, for most of those who are free to choose, the statutory scheme is both cheaper and less risky – dependants are covered 'free' in the statutory scheme and there are restrictions on re-entering the statutory scheme once the right to opt out has been exercised.

SHIFTING COSTS TO PATIENTS

There has been a significant increase in the amount of health care funded directly by patients, either in the form of user charges in the public/private sector or direct payments for services. The direct purchase of services is a significant consequence of rationing policies that exclude services or treatments from cover.

These are significant in the areas of dental care and pharmaceuticals, where drugs may be de-listed (negative list) or else authorised for sale over the counter.

User charges in the public system are a direct result of policy to expand private funding for health services. For example, in Germany the government increased user charges when global budgets were abolished, with the hope of compensating for loss of expenditure control. In Finland and Denmark, user charges were increased following economic recession when national and local funding from taxation was squeezed. There are no randomised control trials of the effect of user charges on utilisation in Europe; most studies trace the effect of a policy change. The evidence from Sweden, France and Denmark does suggest, however, that user charges increase inequalities in access to health care.

Research in Sweden found that in the 1960s high-income groups had higher utilisation of health services. Following a reduction in user fees, results from the 1970s and 1980s showed there were no socio-economic differences in the proportion of the population who visited a doctor, after health status was controlled for. The analysis using data from the 1990s shows the re-emergence of inequalities in utilisation in Sweden favouring the better-off following the major increases in user charges.[21]

In France and Sweden, one in four and one in five people respectively declared they had been put off seeking care for financial reasons. In both countries, women, older people and the unemployed form a large proportion of those not seeking care. Elofsson, Unden and Kradau

---

* Another 2 per cent who are self-employed or public employees have private health insurance.

have shown in the Stockholm area that patient charges were a hindrance to financially and psychosocially disadvantaged groups seeking care. Those who assessed their financial situation as poor were ten times more likely to forego care than those who assessed their financial situation as good.[21,22]

In Denmark, significant increases in user charges for dental care between 1975 and 1990 showed that despite an overall increase in demand, since 1990 household income has been a positive factor in determining the probability for regular dental care, i.e. utilisation was higher at higher incomes.[23] There is little evidence as to how user charges affect health outcomes, but despite the limitations of the research it seems that user charges cause problems for some socio-economic groups in accessing health care services.

CONCLUSIONS

It seems that, at least for the time being, there is a consensus in favour of taxation as the main source of funding for the UK NHS. It has been argued that as long as equity remains of paramount concern, taxation will be favoured over other alternatives.[24] However, experience from the rest of Europe suggests that even when other concerns, such as the economy, are given priority, taxation fares well. Debates in France and Germany centre around the negative impact of social health insurance on the economy. Through the introduction of a health tax and by setting an annual global budget for health, the French state has recently adopted a more interventionist approach. In Germany, the introduction of insurer competition was aimed at reducing contribution rates.

In no country in Europe, with the exception of the Netherlands, does private health insurance account for more than 10 per cent of total health care expenditure. Public policy tends to favour the use of public revenues to ensure universal access to a comprehensive range of services rather than promoting the purchase of private health insurance.

Other countries with traditional welfare approaches to the funding and provision of health care, such as in Scandinavia, did increase the role of user charges. Nonetheless, there is some evidence to show that user charges have acted as a barrier to access, and this policy has attracted criticism and is likely to be reconsidered, at least in Sweden.

If the debate on funding in the UK is closed for the time being (at least until there is a downturn in the economy), we must go beyond questions of how much to spend on health care or how to generate resources. It is also important to examine how the money is spent and what outcomes are achieved.

REFERENCES

1. Jones I M, editor. British Medical Association Advisory Panel. *Health Services Financing.* London: BMA, 1969.
2. Lawson N. *The view from no.11: memoirs of a Tory radical.* London: Bantam Press, 1992.
3. Secretary of State for Health. *The NHS Plan: a plan for investment, a plan for reform.* Cm 4818-I. London: The Stationery Office, 2000.
4. Kanavos P, Mossialos E. International comparisons of health care expenditures: what we know and what we do not know. *Journal of Health Services Research and Policy* 1999; 4 (2): 122–26.
5. OECD. *OECD Health Data 2000: A comparative analysis of 29 countries.* Paris: OECD and CREDES, 2000.

6. BMA Health Policy and Economic Research Unit. *Healthcare funding review.* London: BMA, 2001.

7. Mossialos E *et al.*, editors. *Funding Health Care: options for Europe.* Buckingham: Open University Press, 2001.

8. Mossialos E, Dixon A, McKee M. Paying for the NHS. Editorial. *BMJ* 2000; 320: 197–98.

9. Wagstaff A *et al.* Equity in the finance of health care: some further international comparisons. *Journal of Health Economics* 1999; 18 (3): 263–90.

10. Bouget D. The Juppé Plan and the future of the French social welfare system. *Journal of European Social Policy* 1998; 8 (2): 155–72.

11. Lancry O-J, Sandier S. Recent changes in the financing and provision of medical services in France. *Eurohealth* 1998; 4 (3): 37–39.

12. Clasen J, editor. *Social Insurance in Europe.* Bristol: Policy Press, 1997.

13. Schut F T, van Doorslaer E K. Towards a reinforced agency role of health insurers in Belgium and The Netherlands. *Health Policy* 1999; 48 (1): 47–67.

14. Schut F T. Health care reform in The Netherlands: balancing corporatism, etatism, and market mechanisms. *Journal of Health Politics, Policy and Law* 1995; 20 (3): 615–52.

15. Müller R, Braun B, Grefl S. *Allokative und distributive Effekte von Wettbewerbselementen und Probleme ihrer Implementation in einem sozialen Gesundheitswesen am Beispiel der Erfahrungen in den Niederlanden.* Bremen: University of Bremen, 2000.

16. Normand C, Busse R. Social health insurance. In: Mossialos E *et al.*, editors. *Funding health care: options for Europe.* Buckingham: Open University Press, 2001.

17. Busse R. Health Care Systems in Transition: Germany. In: Dixon A, editor. *Health Care Systems in Transition.* Copenhagen: European Observatory on Health Care Systems, 2000.

18. Zok K. *Anforderungen an die Gesetzliche Krankenversicherung: Einschatzungen und Erwartungen aus Sicht der Versicherten. Vol. 43.* Bonn: Wissenschaftliches Institut der AOK, 1999.

19. Mossialos E, Thomson S. Private health insurance in the European Union. In: Mossialos E *et al.*, editors. *Funding health care: options for Europe.* Buckingham: Open University Press, 2001.

20. Whitehead M, *et al.* As the health divide widens in Sweden and Britain, what's happening to access to care? *BMJ* 1997; 315 (7114): 1006–09.

21. Elofsson S, Unden A L, Krakau I. Patient charges – a hindrance to financially and psychosocially disadvantaged groups seeking care. *Social Science and Medicine* 1998; 46 (10): 1375–80.

22. Petty F. Un français sur quatre renonce aux soins faute d'argent. [One French person out of four fails to seek care for financial reasons.] *Impact Quotidien* 1998: 2.

23. Schwarz E. Changes in utilization and cost sharing within the Danish National Health Insurance dental program, 1975–90. *Acta Odontol Scand* 1996; 54 (1): 29–35.

24. Dixon J. Another healthcare funding review. *BMJ* 2001; 322: 312–13.

The politics of long-term care

Chris Deeming and Justin Keen

INTRODUCTION

It is possible to arrive at two broad political interpretations of the Government's position on long-term care financing. The first is that long-term care financing is in a mess and has not been properly thought through within the context of the welfare system. In essence, the Government is confused about its application of principles such as affordability, efficiency and equity. The second interpretation is that the Government's position is based upon ideas whose time has come, and developments in long-term care financing are congruent with developments in other areas of social policy. In other words, the Government has a coherent agenda for welfare reform that stresses the rights and responsibilities of individuals and the importance of a mixed economy for welfare finance and provision. Within this position individuals are encouraged to make adequate provision for their future, leaving the State to target resources at only the very poorest members of society.

It is not clear which of these two interpretations is the more accurate because the debate since the Royal Commission report has been preoccupied with the definition of 'nursing care'. This relatively narrow debate has, however, been rather helpful in exposing the ideology underpinning the Government's and Royal Commission's positions. It is a debate that has been brought into sharper focus with the recent decision of the Scottish Executive. While the reforms in long-term care could be seen as consistent with general trends in the Government's welfare policy, after the Scottish decision many debates that the Government would prefer had run their course are relevant once again.

The technical debate about the definition of nursing care will be resolved, but the wider political debate is unlikely to be settled in the short term. There are two possible outcomes of this wider debate. Either the Government will ride the wave of interest-group discontent and stick to its belief in means-testing personal care, or public pressure in England and Wales, initiated by interest groups and spurred on by the possibility of free personal care in Scotland, will force a U-turn. The former is the more likely, but if the latter is the case, the Government will be forced to reconsider its ideological stance in order to arrive at a more politically acceptable system of long-term care financing.

In this paper we explore these two scenarios. We consider some of the policy options open to the Government if it is provided with the opportunity to rethink the financing of long-term care – what might a fairer system look like? We also consider an unchanged Government position in England and Wales. We ask how the English and Welsh financing system could work efficiently and effectively for individuals, and consider some of the major tensions that will need addressing. We begin, though, by outlining the current status of the long-term care financing debate and the issues of affordability and equity.

THE CURRENT LONG-TERM CARE DEBATE

IS PERSONAL CARE AFFORDABLE?

Under the Government's proposed financing system,[1] individuals living in England and Wales who need residential care will be responsible for their 'hotel costs' (housing and living costs) and for the costs of their personal care. Those with adequate means will be required to pay. Individuals will no longer be responsible for the cost of nursing care – the NHS, and ultimately the tax-payer, will foot the bill. The provision of free nursing care has been widely welcomed.

The Government in England and the Assembly in Wales have decided not to implement one of the main recommendations of the Royal Commission on Long Term Care – that personal care costs should be met by the State subject to an assessment of need of care.[2] The Government, following the line of the 'minority report' (the 'Note of Dissent' written by two of the Commissioners, Joel Joffe and David Lipsey[3]) claimed that free personal care did not represent the best use of available resources. The Government's decision to make a distinction between free nursing care and means-tested personal care has provoked much criticism from interest groups, partly on principle and partly on

the practicalities of finding a workable definition of nursing care.

The Government claims that it is facing hard choices within a fixed budget. Intermediate care is the Government's preferred option, at a cost of nearly £1 billion over four years. It views free personal care as a less efficient use of resources. The costs of personal care were estimated in the Royal Commission report to be around £1.1 billion per year (rising to £6 billion by 2051). The minority Commissioners disputed these estimates, arguing that setting a zero price for personal care would inflate demand, and hence costs. The implication was that such a policy would be unaffordable. In turn, of course, the estimates in the minority Commissioners' report can be challenged – as they have been by Age Concern.[4]

In the context of universal access to free personal care, 'unaffordability' is in fact used euphemistically: it is not so much the scale of the *financial costs* to the Exchequer that is important, but the *opportunity costs* in terms of forgone benefits in spending limited resources in some other way. Essentially, the minority Commissioners and the Government take the view that these forgone benefits are greater than the benefits to be derived from free personal care. In other words, the argument hinges on views about allocative efficiency.

Considerations of allocative efficiency are not merely technical, but will necessarily involve judgements about the fairness of the distribution of benefits (and costs) across different groups in society. The next section considers the equity principles that underpin the financing of long-term care.

EQUITY: THE CORE OF THE DEBATE

The focus on the distinction between free nursing care and free personal care has had important consequences for the long-term care debate. To many it has appeared that the problem is whether or not a workable definition of nursing care can be identified. But this has distracted attention from an examination of certain principles, in particular, equity, which lie at the heart of much of the disagreements over long-term care.

In fact, fairness has been stated by ministers as a guiding criterion for long-term care. In a speech in the House of Commons in December 1999, Alan Milburn stated that: 'We shall base any future reforms ... on three key principles: choice, fairness and quality ... just as elsewhere in our welfare reform programme, our policy will be that people should provide for themselves whenever they are able to do so.'[5]

In practice, the problem is complicated by the fact that the Royal Commission and Government turn out to be arguing about the consistency of each others' positions, rather than about fundamental equity principles. The result is that the principles at stake are somewhat obscured.

One approach to the concept of equity is to distinguish between two dimensions: horizontal and vertical equity The former is most usually invoked in terms of *provision* or *access* to care. So, horizontal equity implies that equals (in terms of *health care needs*) are treated equally. In contrast, vertical equity is usually applied to the equity of *financing* of care and implies that unequals (in terms of *income*) are treated unequally. In other words, vertical equity suggests that the well off should contribute more towards the costs

of health care than the less well off. (How much more is paid – that is, the degree of inequity favouring the poor – is a matter of social policy; currently, the UK tax system – which largely funds the NHS – is mildly progressive – the rich pay proportionately more than the poor.) Overall, and in comparison with many other countries, the NHS is fairly equitable, both in terms of provision (or access) and financing. The problem in long-term care, however, is that it is perceived to be unfair along both dimensions of finance and provision.

All key stakeholders in long-term care agree that nursing care should be free at the point of delivery, irrespective of setting. This has the effect of making the provision of nursing care more equitable – in effect, *extending* the principle of equity of provision from the NHS out into all long-term care settings, including nursing homes. But this extension of equity is not costless. In particular, universal free nursing care means that those whom some may feel can afford to pay directly for their own care enjoy free access – arguably (and within a fixed budget) at the expense of the poor. In one sense this could be seen as inequitable if the needs of the poor are not completely satisfied as a result of free access by the rich. Of course, such a 'cost' of universal free access is generally thought worth bearing in most aspects of NHS provision.

The majority Commissioners and critics of the Government argue that the principle of free universal access should be extended further to include personal care (irrespective of where care is provided). However, in rejecting this, the Government invoked the argument that part of the cost of such universal access would be that the rich benefited at the expense of the poor. In other words, personal care should be paid for by those who can afford it, so that the State's resources can be better targeted at people who are most in need. It would appear that the minority Commissioners and the Government are prepared to tolerate continuing inconsistencies in current patterns of provision of health and social care, and face accusations of unfairness. As Lipsey and Joffe stated: 'Just because health care is free it does not follow that personal care should be free too. There is no principle that just because one thing is free, something else should be free.'[3]

The debate is not just about equity principles but also about consistency, particularly consistency with other decisions concerning access to nursing care. While the Government accept the notion that nursing care should be free to all and in all settings, and also acknowledge that this will *differentially benefit* people with higher incomes and assets financially, they argue that personal care should be paid for by those who can afford it, in order that people with higher incomes and assets are *no better off* than they are now (because they already have to pay for it).

The Government and the minority Commissioners do not offer any reasons or explanations as to why personal care should be considered to be fundamentally different (and hence subject to means-testing) in one setting (nursing homes, for example) but not in another (for example, an NHS hospital). Moreover, there is little public support for this distinction. Evidence suggests that public, in time of need, look to the State for care,[6,7] that they are generally against means-testing,[8] and that most do not distinguish between care settings when asked questions about free provision of personal care (King's Fund unpublished data).

All of this suggests that we must shift the spotlight to the majority Commissioners' position and examine their arguments for consistency. The minority Commissioners refer to a table of aids and adaptations produced by the majority Commissioners in Appendix 1 of the main report.[2] The table shows that the majority Commissioners believe that some items on the list should be provided free while others should be means-tested, even though both are provided by occupational therapists. The minority Commissioners use this observation to claim that the majority Commissioners' general position is also inconsistent.

Of course, this particular charge of inconsistency cannot be used to support the minority Commissioners' stance on distinguishing between nursing and personal care (unless two wrongs *do* make a right) any more than the fact that the NHS make direct patient charges for prescriptions, dentistry, etc. As has been demonstrated, these charges can have deleterious effects on access and health, issues acknowledged by the Government in its dental strategy.[9]

It is important to stress that within a complicated issue there is further complication. Concerns about equity and consistency are intersected by another debate concerning the *scope* of the policy area over which a particular principle should apply. For example, the majority Commissioners focused on such issues as nursing and personal care, while the Government has sought to create a trade-off between personal care and intermediate care. The two sides are defining the scope of the debate in different ways. This serves, in practice, to further confuse an already confused debate.

While both sides have appealed to consistency arguments – and both have failed to different degrees – consistency cannot be a policy end in itself. For instance, neither side appears concerned about the equity implications of maintaining the *status quo* by means-testing hotel costs (which are free in the NHS settings).

Given concerns about the Government's decision on funding long-term care, where now? Is it possible to plot some future changes that might help to address these concerns?

A RETHINK ON LONG-TERM CARE FINANCING

Despite the Government's decisions on long-term care funding, it is conceivable that they may need to reconsider. We have argued that decisions made north of the border make this more likely in England and Wales. If a rethink is possible, we suspect that the Government will face some of the options it originally faced between March 1999 (when the Royal Commission report was published) and July 2000 (when it formally responded to it).

The most equitable and efficient policy solution is one that pools risk across society and redistributes resources according to need, as the majority Commissioners argued. Universal or near universal schemes remove individual financial risks associated with long-term care. If this is accepted, then how should this be done and what should be covered? There are two main methods: general taxation and social insurance, and both can offer varying degrees of coverage.

A truly *universal* model would require that all the costs of long-term care (both care and 'hotel costs') would be paid collectively (and in practice, from general taxation). In effect, it would be an expansion of NHS provision (though need not be part of the NHS). This was dismissed by the Royal Commissioners as being undesirable and unnecessary – an improper use of public funds, and therefore an unrealistic option. The majority Commissioners proposed a variation of this model, with access to care free at the point of delivery and means-testing for 'hotel costs'.

One alternative is to move to a system of social insurance. Such schemes also pool risk and, depending on how they are designed, may or may not offer universal coverage. Whatever the design, qualifying for benefits depends upon having made a required level of contributions during one's working life. Essentially there are three types of social insurance: pay as you go (PAYG), funded, and partial social insurance. A PAYG scheme offers insurance cover for today's elderly financed by today's tax-payer. Therefore, it redistributes from today's tax-payers to those who would today have to fund their own care and to the beneficiaries of their wills – typically the better-off elderly. A funded social insurance scheme does not have the kind of distributional consequences identified with the PAYG alternative. Individuals pay a sum from their income and this would be invested on their behalf in order to provide a fund from which future long-term care needs would be financed. The main problem is the transitional cost: it may take up to a generation before the fund is sufficient to provide comprehensive cover.

A partial social insurance scheme would follow the pattern of the previous models, but insurance would only cover the care component of long-term care costs. 'Hotel costs' would be means-tested. A variation on this is social insurance for personal care only, with the NHS (tax-payer) funding nursing care, and 'hotel costs' means-tested. The Government position is, at least conceptually, reasonably close to this option. It could choose to offer a partial social insurance scheme for personal care rather than leave it to the market. The main problem with any social insurance scheme is the inevitable creation of a two-tier system. Since coverage is not universal, the safety net provided by the State is likely to be of a lower standard than that provided through the social insurance scheme.

AN UNCHANGED POSITION IN ENGLAND AND WALES

WILL THE GOVERNMENT'S PRESCRIPTION WORK?

Although a reconsideration by the Government of its decisions is possible, in the short term, however, it is more likely that the decisions will be implemented. But how will the new arrangements work in practice? Below, we examine two issues: the extent to which individuals can afford to pay for long-term care in the way the Government expects, and the incentives to them to save more than they do at present.

If individuals cannot contribute the amounts that the Government expects, then its prescription will not work, either for today's pensioners who are required to pay for personal care or for those currently of working age, who are being encouraged to take more financial responsibility for their old age. An important aspect of the new arrangements is an expectation that people of working age, particularly those on average and below-average incomes, will make adequate provision for themselves in order to ensure a reasonable standard of living in later life. The Government has been considering ways in which long-term care savings or insurance products can be made more attractive. At the same time, it is also encouraging people to invest in a second pension.[10] This leads to an obvious question: will people on average and below-average incomes be able to afford to invest in supplementary pensions and long-term care savings or insurance products? Evidence suggests that this is unlikely for most people and that the majority will therefore find it difficult to avoid a means-tested old age.[6,11] Moreover, many of today's pensioners on average and below-average incomes struggle to afford care services in domestic settings and may not be receiving the care they need.[6,12]

The ability of individuals to afford long-term care, and the absence of credible incentives to set aside adequate savings, suggests that the Government has not properly thought through the links, and interaction, between some policies. Notably, it has not linked social security and long-term care policies from the point of view of individuals and family units. In this sense, the debate about long-term care funding has been too narrowly focused, for example, upon the extent to which people should be responsible for the costs of their own care, with some advocating the benefits of free universal care and others the benefits of greater targeting of scarce resources on the most needy by means-testing personal care.

Figure 1: Long-term care is caught at the intersection between three main areas of social policy

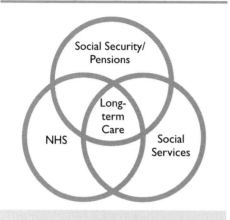

The separate debate over pensions has focused on the method of increasing pensioner incomes, with some arguing for an increase in incomes for all pensioners by restoring the link to earnings, while others defend the current system of relating pension increases to prices and the reliance on means-testing to ensure a basic minimum (the Minimum Income Guarantee). In practice, though, decisions in one area of policy can have major implications for others. Long-term care is at the interface between three major policy areas with somewhat separate financing and delivery structures, and the interaction between these areas of policy needs to be fully considered if the system is to work efficiently (see Figure 1).

Long-term care policy, and similarly pensions policy, have developed in a piecemeal fashion over many years. Long-term care, in particular, has been subject to a great deal of incremental change, at times originating in other parts of the Welfare State, but little consideration has

been given to the aggregate effect on the system of many separate changes. We have argued for a much broader view of the issues and suggest a more holistic approach to considering the financing of long-term care – one that is firmly based around the individual.

WHERE NOW?

The NHS Plan constitutes the Government's blueprint for the service over the next ten years and, as such, individuals in England and Wales will be responsible for funding personal care and 'hotel costs'. If tomorrow's pensioners are to avoid a means-tested old age then the Government will need to develop a coherent policy framework that works for individuals. There appear to be two main options on offer: equity release and private savings/insurance.

EQUITY RELEASE

Unlocking housing equity offers the potential to help pay for old age. For example, the proposal to disregard house values during the first three months in a care home may do much to prevent premature decisions to sell property and to enable individuals to return home after a period of recuperation and rehabilitation. It is expected that some 30,000 people a year may benefit from this. But the use of housing equity has much wider potential than merely helping to pay for residential care, however. Equity-release mechanisms could supplement income, raise money for capital needs and generally improve quality of life. Taken alone, this may not be a solution to the financing of old age, but it could be part of the answer for some people. It is not clear what impact Government proposals, which came into effect on 1 April, will have on the equity-release market or the Government's own version of the equity-release scheme. £85 million will be invested in this over the next three years.

But is this enough? Currently there is no regulation, and there are anomalies in the way income from equity release relates to social security. A recent report on equity-release mechanisms recommended that the equivalent of pensioner credit for people with income just above the MIG should be extended to income from equity-release mechanisms.[13] If this can be made to work, and hence create better opportunities for individuals to take greater financial responsibility for their old age, this would allow the Government to target the very needy – the income and asset poor.

SAVINGS/INSURANCE

The Government has been considering the possibilities for savings and insurance products with the financial services industry. There are two other broad options in this area of policy: free-standing private insurance and special private savings accounts. Free-standing private long-term care insurance exists today but has not really developed. By itself it is not an option, as it depends on pooling risk on a voluntary basis and therefore requires adverse selection to be absent or screened out by the insurer. Better regulation and public education may help the market develop further, but take-up of these policies is likely to be extremely limited (as it is even in the US market).

Saving for long-term care is not an efficient option for individuals. Not everyone will need long-term care, therefore it would be unrealistic and socially inefficient for everyone to save to meet the average cost of needing care, let alone the maximum cost.

A BALANCE BETWEEN TWO PRINCIPLES

Government policy appears caught between two principles – the 'rainy-day principle' and the 'cascade principle'. Under the first principle, people are encouraged to take responsibility for themselves; under the second, people save not just for a rainy day, but also because they want their assets to cascade down to the next generation.

The Government, on the one hand, appear to want wealth to be passed down the generations (the 'cascade principle'). For example, the three-month housing disregard is expected to benefit 30,000 people a year and the asset disregard has also been raised to £18,000. On the other hand, the Government is encouraging people to take more responsibility for the possibility of their needing long-term care and confiscating the savings and assets of people who need long-term care.

Has the Government achieved the right balance between these two principles? This seems unlikely, Although the Government's long-term care financing policy may be welcomed in many respects, such incremental policy changes are unlikely to be sustainable in the long term as there are too may tensions and inconsistencies contained within current policies.

CONCLUSION

The long-term care financing debate so far has had the appearance of a technical dispute, which, to some extent it is. However, it involves a much broader political disagreement about the role of the State and the boundary between public and private responsibilities in long-term care.

In terms of the particulars, the claim that certain aspects of long-term care are 'unaffordable' hinge not on empirical evidence but on value judgements concerning priorities. Moreover, the decision to make a distinction between nursing care and personal care has redefined the definition of the public and the private responsibilities for financing long-term care – the right to free nursing care paid for by the State and continued private responsibility for personal care. The Government has maintained that this is fair, but this view is arguable.

The dispute over universal access to free personal care can be thought of as a difference in emphasis of the importance of equity of finance (the Government) and of access (the majority Commissioners). The debate is not easily resolved because a number of complicated equity considerations are inter-linked, both within long-term care and other areas of public and private life such as health care and pensions. Given this, it is important to think through the links between long-term care, pensions and other policies from the point of view of the individual and household.

In addition, efficiency may be jeopardised under the Government's decision on long-term care funding due to weak incentives for individuals to save for their personal long-term care costs later in life. Furthermore, a complex system has been made even more complicated as a result of the Government's decisions on long-term care. We argue that it is not so much that mixed financing strategies do not work efficiently, more that the mix offered by the Government appears to be particularly unsatisfactory.

Over the long term, the decision taken by the Government on long-term care

financing is unlikely to be sustainable as it introduces new complexities and areas of potential dispute, as well as failing to satisfy demands from the public. The Government may ultimately have to rethink its policies in this area.[14,15] If so, it could do worse than to consider a system of finance that pools risk across society and redistributes resources according to need. In practice, the use of general taxation as the source of funding is likely to be more acceptable than social insurance in the UK.

REFERENCES

1. Department of Health. *The NHS Plan: The Government's response to the Royal Commission on Long Term Care*. London: The Stationery Office, 2000.
2. Royal Commission on Long Term Care. *With respect to old age*. London: The Stationery Office, 1999.
3. Royal Commission on Long Term Care: Note of Dissent. *With respect to old age*. Cm 4192-I. London: The Stationery Office, 1999: 113–43.
4. Age Concern. *The future of health and care of older people: The best is yet to come*. The millennium papers. London: Age Concern, 1999.
5. Milburn A. *House of Commons Hansard 1999*; 2 December.
6. Deeming C, Keen K. *Paying for old age?* London: King's Fund, 2000.
7. Parker G, Clarke H. Will you need me, will you still feed me? – Paying for care in old age. *Social Policy and Administration* 1997; 31 (2).
8. Department of Social Security. *Attitudes to the welfare state and the response to reform*. Research Report no. 88. Leeds: Department of Social Security, 1999.
9. Department of Health. *Modernising NHS dentistry – implementing the NHS Plan*. London: The Stationery Office, 2000.
10. Department of Social Security. *A new*

contract for welfare: partnership in pensions. London: DSS, 1998.

11. Rake *et al.* British Pension Policy in the Twenty-first Century: a partnership in pensions or a marriage to the means-test? *Social Policy and Administration* 2000; 34 (3): 296–317.

12. Evandrou M, Falkingham J. The personal social services. In: Glennerster H, Hills J, eds. *The state of welfare: the economics of social spending.* Oxford: Oxford University Press, 1998.

13. The Actuarial Profession. *Report on Equity Release Mechanisms.* January 2001.

14. Hargreaves I, Christie I. Rethinking retirement. In: Hargreaves I, Christie I. *Tomorrow's Politics: The Third Way.* London: Demos, 1998.

15. Giddens A. *The Third Way: The renewal of social democracy.* Oxford: Polity Press, 1998.

Health Act flexibilities: first steps*

Liisa Kurunmäki, Peter Miller and Justin Keen

INTRODUCTION

'Joined-up working' is the battle cry for the current government in its attempts to encourage a further stage in the modernisation of public services.[1] 'Flexibility' is the name given to attempts to facilitate such a policy by encouraging partnership working among service providers.[2] Section 31 of the Health Act 1999 gave considerable prominence to these issues by introducing powers to enable different forms of partnership arrangements: *pooled budgets* allowed health and social services to bring together some resources into a joint budget; *lead commissioning* allowed one authority – either health care or social services – to take responsibility for commissioning services; and *integrated provision* allowed an NHS Trust or Primary Care Trust to provide social care services, thus offering integrated services from one provider rather than many. *The NHS Plan*[3] gave added impetus to this policy. It made partnership working between health and social care appear to be a necessity rather than an option.

These recent developments pose significant challenges for professionals and managers at all levels within health and social care agencies. Issues of financial control, governance and accountability become focal points in an interprofessional encounter that is already inherent with tensions. New organisational forms seem to be required, along with new ways of managing the delivery of vital services. Those charged with managing and working within such new entities have to address often fundamental procedural and policy issues.

At a procedural level, the first issue to address is whether to make use of the Health Act powers at all, or whether to continue with existing and largely informal co-operative working. Those that decide to experiment with the new flexibilities are faced with a choice between different types of partnership, and have to weigh up the benefits of each. They have to choose whether to opt initially for what might appear as the less-demanding mechanism of lead commissioning, or whether to take the bolder step of opting for pooled budgets or integrated provision at the outset. A

* The study has been funded by the Institute of Chartered Accountants in England and Wales, and the King's Fund. Their support is gratefully acknowledged.

further possibility to consider is that of opting for a combination of, say, pooled budgets and integrated or lead commissioning. There is also the issue of choosing which services and user groups to begin with, and whether there are synergies to be obtained among them, which might imply experimenting initially with more than one service. The actors have to make these fundamental choices, mindful of the need to continue to improve levels of service delivery, while seeking to persuade those at all levels of the hierarchy of the merits of partnership working.

At a policy level, the actors have to define at the outset, and in writing, the aims, intended outcomes and targets of the partnership. They have to specify what resources will be shared and what level of sharing is desirable. They have to decide whether to include other agencies and individuals, such as carers, schools, housing associations, and so forth. They have to devise and apply eligibility criteria for specified services, create mechanisms for appeals, and ensure that such criteria and mechanisms are acceptable to all partners. The compatibility between the proposed partnership arrangements and existing policies such as Health Improvement Programmes (HImPs), Best Value plans and the like has to be documented. And, once up and running, agreement has to be reached on a wide and complex range of governance arrangements, including meeting accountability, performance monitoring, inspection and audit requirements, even where the accounting years and VAT regimes of the partners vary.

This article continues by providing some of the background to these issues. It then describes a research project examining early examples of partnership working in five different areas, and concludes by noting some of the policy issues raised.

BACKGROUND

Formal policies for the joint financing and delivery of health and social care have had a long, and often problematic, history.[4] Policy-makers have worked on the premise that co-ordination of commissioning and delivery of services can and should be better than it is. They have, however, had to operate within a system that has imposed clear demarcations between health and social care in both the financing and delivery of services. This has tended to limit the effectiveness of initiatives down the years, and experiences have been mixed.

After Labour came to power in 1997, 'partnership' became a key term in the social policy lexicon. There emerged a new impetus to erode the boundaries between health and social care. A range of initiatives sought to encourage innovative cross-sectoral working. Recent examples include Joint Investment Plans (JIPs), Health Improvement Programmes, Partnership Grants, and the Better Government for Older People programme. The Labour Government also promoted other types of partnerships. For example, it vigorously promoted public–private partnerships. It inherited the Private Finance Initiative from the Conservatives, and has developed and used it in the NHS and elsewhere. Labour has also initiated new multi-agency approaches to health improvement in Health Action Zones. The result is that different types of partnership working are being implemented by service providers alongside one another. Every locality has to have a HImP and a JIP, and may be working on PFI, intermediate care, and other initiatives. Partnership is everywhere.

The Health Act 1999 removes the constraints on joint working at all levels.[5] It provides a statutory framework for joint financing of health and social care, and embraces other types of partnership working. For example, the Government has indicated that intermediate care is an area where it welcomes the use of private finance, whether through the Private Finance Initiative or other forms of contract. Pooled or integrated budget arrangements could, in principle, be used to co-ordinate the use of resources for both capital and ongoing financing of intermediate care.

It is not possible to predict whether pooled and integrated budgets will run into the same problems experienced in the past, or whether the new budgetary arrangements will lead to new possibilities – and problems. The NHS and social services departments have distinct budgetary, legal and cultural histories. These histories will not disappear quickly, even within new institutional structures. Equally, and alongside the potential benefits of the flexibilities offered by the Health Act, formal partnership arrangements may impose different requirements and alter already established co-operative systems, undermining good local practices. In short, the only way of identifying the potential and the problems of partnership working is to go into the field.

RESEARCH ISSUES

The principal aim of the project is to examine the first steps towards partnership working being taken by a range of different authorities. Our focus is particularly on the governance,

performance management and accountability issues raised by the partnership arrangements. But we address these issues within the wider context of a concern with the interprofessional issues raised by seeking to create formal co-operative mechanisms for health, social care, and other agencies to work together. We are looking at a range of different specialisms, including learning disabilities, child care and elderly people. We selected a range of different geographical areas, albeit spread across southern England. By entering the field when the sites are commencing their experiments, we hope to be able to capture the process by which partnership working develops.

Our concern is to study such policies and practices 'in the making', while NHS and social service providers confront the ambiguities, opportunities and procedural difficulties of partnership working in all its various forms. Rather than arriving after the event, when things are well established, we wish to document and analyse the complexities of such a reform process as local participants seek to make it work. We seek to understand the factors that facilitate or hinder the introduction of formal partnership arrangements, their perceived benefits, and the perceptions and reactions of different stakeholders to them. Through a combination of semi-structured interviews with different participants, observation of meetings, and analysis of relevant documentation, we are examining developments in selected sites between now and early Summer 2001. The study does not aspire to comprehensiveness or completeness. The aim is to identify some of the issues faced by a small number of service providers in this uncertain and rapidly changing world.

It is too early in the study to offer even a preliminary summary of our findings, but it is possible to identify some of the specific research issues that are coming to the fore as we progress. The issue of informal co-operation prior to the take-up of formal partnership arrangements is likely to be of considerable interest, and we hope to find out whether this is one of the pre-conditions for the success of formal partnerships. We are also interested to see whether some sites decide that they can achieve the much-vaunted flexibility and co-operation promoted in the Health Act without invoking its formal procedures and policies. We are particularly interested in the local mechanisms and forums for co-operation, information sharing and apportioning of resources devised by the various actors as partnership working develops. These may help us to understand not only how and why partnership working succeeds, but may also offer some models for learning by other sites.

The development of performance monitoring mechanisms acceptable to all parties also looks likely to be a significant and challenging issue for partnerships, to the extent that health and social care agencies have different traditions in this respect. We will be interested to find out whether there is a common sequence to the take-up of partnership arrangements, with lead commissioning typically being the first step. Also, if this proves to be the case, we will attempt to ascertain the timescale for moving to pooled budgets, and whether they are an immediate or medium-term objective. More generally, we will be seeking to explore whether there are any major concerns for either health care or social care agencies regarding the overall direction of current policies, and the implications for either

party in the partnership. In another national setting, the emergence of a 'hybrid' entity has been noted,[6] and we are particularly keen to see how the issues of boundaries is addressed in this formal encounter between health and social agencies in the UK.

POLICY CHALLENGES

The numerous attempts by the Government to advance partnership working indicate the strength of the desire to weaken the boundaries between health and social care. The increasing efforts of individual actors and agencies to develop co-operative working at a local level parallel and reinforce the current direction of Government policy. But policies often overlap, and do not always harmonise perfectly. JIPs, HImPs and longer-established commissioning arrangements have to be synchronised with the recently-proposed Health Act flexibilities, and these in turn have to be aligned with such policies as those concerning intermediate care, and the recently published *NHS Plan*, which sets out the concept of Care Trusts. Even if one policy supplants another over time, those who have to deliver services are in an almost perpetual transitional phase. New policies often appear even while the mechanisms and details of earlier ones are only just being devised. The issue of integrating or harmonising policies is perhaps one of the longest-standing challenges facing not only policy-makers, but also those who have to put the policies to work.

Trust is another fundamental issue, and has both a personal and an institutional dimension. At a personal level, the lead commissioner or pooled fund manager has to be trusted by the various participants in the partnership. The level of contributions to a pooled budget, and even its very existence, are likely to be affected significantly by the degree of trust. At an institutional level, it is important that policies such as integrated provision or Care Trusts are not perceived as allowing or encouraging the possibility of takeover by one partner or another.

Relatedly, the varying and possibly conflicting norms of agencies such as health and social services, as well as education and housing, need to be considered. While policies aspire to convergence or co-operation, existing norms can run counter to these aims. Whether the norms concern basic principles of care and treatment, rights to care, the funding of care, performance targets, or much broader issues of professional identity, the differing norms of the participating partners can prove challenging for policy-makers intent on eroding the boundaries between service providers.

One further issue worth noting concerns the long-term aspirations of policy-makers. The past decade or so has seen an increasing emphasis on co-operation or partnership in all its forms. Current policies are, if anything, seeking to speed up and strengthen these developments. But if integration is the goal, some fundamental issues of accountability, responsibility and performance evaluation will have to be faced. If services are to be delivered from a single point, yet financial accountability remains at least dual, integration may well encounter limits earlier rather than later. If performance targets are nationally set, and if these are specific to each of the partners, once again this may constrain the development of partnership arrangements. In the longer run, if the purchase of new buildings is required, and

if these are to be jointly owned, then the issue of financial accountability will become even more prominent an issue. These are important issues, and it would be a pity if they proved to be a stumbling block when co-operation is genuinely desired by the various actors and agencies involved in both policy formulation and service provision.

To identify some of the policy challenges facing partnership working is not an indication of pessimism concerning the Health Act flexibilities; quite the reverse. Even though it is too early in the project to offer even tentative conclusions, it is clear that important innovations are occurring. Existing modes of informal co-operation are, in a number of interesting cases, being transformed into formal partnership arrangements. The flexibilities of the Health Act are being used, even if there is still a long way to go. Policies and services are being integrated, trust is developing, and the differences between the norms of the partners are being addressed. It is important to identify both the achievements and the hurdles that remain. And it is important that local experiences and experiments are built upon and learned from. For it is these that will tell us how far, and how fast, it is possible to proceed with the new Health Act flexibilities.

REFERENCES

1. *Modernising Government*. Cm 4310; March 1999; *Modernising Social Services: Promoting independence, improving protection, raising standards*. Cm 4169; November 1998; *The New NHS: Modern, dependable*. Cm 3807; December 1997.

2. Department of Health. *Partnership in action: new opportunities for joint working between health and social services*. Discussion

document. Department of Health, 1998.

3. Secretary of State for Health. *The NHS Plan: a plan for investment, a plan for reform.* Cm 4818-I. London: The Stationery Office, 2000.

4. Bridgen P, Lewis J. *Elderly People and the Boundary between Health and Social Care 1946–1991: whose responsibility?* London: Nuffield Trust, 1999.

5. Glendinning C, Clarke J. Old Wine, New Bottles? Prospects for NHS/local authority partnerships under 'New Labour'. Paper given at the ESRC seminar on *The Third Way in Public Services – partnership.* York: April 2000.

6. Kurunmäki L. A *Hybrid Profession: the appropriation of management accounting expertise by medical professionals.* London: LSE Health, Discussion Papers in Health Policy No. 18, 2000.

NHS spending: the wrong target (again)?

John Appleby and Seán Boyle

It is a year since the Prime Minister revealed during a Sunday morning TV interview that he intended to raise total health care spending (by increasing public spending) to match the average proportion of GDP spent in the rest of the European Union.

Most commentators agreed that Tony Blair's calculations of the overall EU share spent on health care were just 'plain wrong'.[1,2] Moreover, the financial feasibility of setting such a target had not been thought through, nor, indeed, had the sense in setting such a target in the first place. With new data from the OECD, it is clear that over the next few years UK spending on health care will remain significantly below the average of other European Union countries.

CALCULATING AN AVERAGE

Despite all the evidence to the contrary, the Government still seems convinced that it has done enough to lever UK health care spending into the middle of the EU pack. Towards the end of 2000,

the Health Secretary Alan Milburn, in evidence to the House of Commons Health Committee, returned to the fray. According to Milburn, it is the experts that are mistaken, and the figure the UK should be aiming for is 8 per cent of GDP – a figure that Milburn reckons will be achieved.

At the Health Committee, Milburn confirmed that the Government's choice of target for EU average spend was the arithmetic mean. In other words, the percentage health care spends in each EU country were simply summed and divided by the number of EU countries (15, including the UK). That is, for the mathematically inclined:

$$\frac{1}{15} \times \sum_{i=1}^{15} \left(\frac{h_i}{g_i}\right) \times 100$$

Where h_i = total spending on health care for country i, and g_i = total GDP, both measured in US$ purchasing power parities

For 1998, this gives an arithmetic average of 7.99 per cent for the average spend on health care for all EU countries, or 8.08 per cent if the UK is excluded. But the implication of this calculation is that *equal weight* is given to each country in the EU regardless of size of population or wealth. While there is no mathematical justification for this,* there may be a political justification in as much that EU member states are treated equally in most spheres of EU life.

The question is, however, whether such an egalitarian view of the *politics* and practices of the EU should, in the case of *statistics* about average percentage health care spend, override the straightforward mathematics of calculating an average.

If a health care spending target based on the average spend of our European neighbours is felt to be the right aspirational goal, then it would be better to leave to one side the machinations of European politics and calculate an average which, treating the EU as one large country, corresponds to average spend per EU citizen. This would mean calculating a *weighted* average. A plausible weight would be GDP. Again, for the mathematically inclined:

$$\left(\frac{\sum\limits_{i=1}^{15}(h_i)}{\sum\limits_{i=1}^{15}(g_i)} \right) \times 100$$

Where h_i = total spending on health care for country i, and g_i = total GDP, both measured in US$ purchasing power parities

For 1998, this calculation of the weighted average gives a figure of 8.66 per cent if the UK is included or 9.03 per cent if it is excluded – 0.67 per cent and 0.95 per cent higher respectively than the arithmetic means preferred by the Department of Health.

We would argue, as we have elsewhere,[1] that this method of calculating the average makes more sense and does not require the somewhat convoluted political justification which seems to underlie Government thinking.

However, even if it is accepted that there are alternative and legitimate ways of counting the number of angels that can fit on a pin head, the Prime Minister's spending pledge raises a number of further issues:

- the comparability of OECD health spend and GDP figures collected and collated from individual countries
- how health care spending will change over the next few years (that is, where will the target be by the end of the next Parliament?)
- was the Prime Minister's suggested target the right one to choose in the first place?

COMPARABILITY

While the OECD has tried to ensure that the figures it compiles for its health database are comparable, there are known anomalies.[3] We do not intend to delve too deeply into this here. Some of the issues that have received attention are: the inclusion of nursing home spending (the reported UK figure for total health

---

* Of course, one strange result of using the arithmetic mean in this case is that if it is then multiplied by the total GDP for all EU countries the resulting figure for total health care spending in the EU is less than the actual figure! This is hardly a common-sense understanding of an average.

care spending does not include it, but a number of other EU countries do);[2] the construction of appropriate indices of purchasing power parity (PPP); the treatment of taxation; and levels of informal care. Other differences may also exist (including some that may affect the comparability of the GDP data set held by the OECD).

Without detailed investigation it is difficult to compensate for such data problems. However, the probability that the figures are not wholly comparable needs to be borne in mind (although we suspect that these problems are unlikely to overturn the analysis and conclusions below).

FUTURE HEALTH CARE SPENDING

However the average EU spend is calculated, it is certainly not a static target. Figure 1 – based on the latest OECD health data set for 2000 – shows the inexorable rising share of national wealth consumed by health care in the EU and the UK since the 1960s.

The figure shows two lines for the average EU health care spend – one based on the Department's preferred measure of the arithmetic mean, and the other based on a weighted average. Linear time trend projections* for both averages have been made to 2006.

UK spending figures for the years 2000–03 are based on the Government's actual spending plans for the NHS[4] plus private spending (estimated to be a constant 1.1 per cent of GDP for each year). UK spending for the years 2004–06 are estimates based on the average annual real terms increase in NHS spending over

Figure 1: Total health care spending as a proportion of GDP: actual and projected

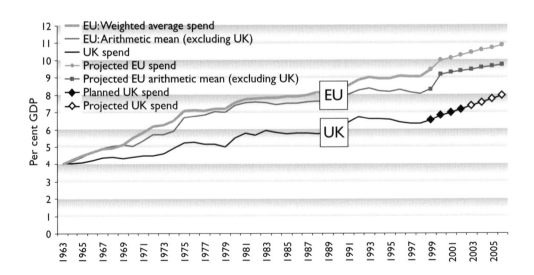

* A linear trend fits the EU data well. Some non-linear estimates were tried but offered little extra explanatory power.

the years 1999–2003 (i.e. 6.1 per cent), again with the addition of private spending of 1.1 per cent of GDP. The GDP figures for the UK for the years 1999–2006 are based on Treasury data and forecasts.[5]

The chart is interesting for a number of reasons. The most obvious is the gap between the UK and the rest of the EU in terms of average proportion of GDP spent on health care.

While Blair suggested that New Labour's aspiration was to close this gap, it is evident from projecting the EU average that, despite the extra billions promised in last year's budget, the (moving) target will be missed.

In terms of the EU weighted average, by the putative end of the next Parliament in 2006, the UK will remain significantly below the rest of the EU – which, at nearly 11 per cent, is somewhat higher than the Government's figure of 8 per cent. In fact the rest of the EU is already spending 9 per cent of its GDP on health care. At this rate the gap between us and the rest will only return to what it was in 1999.

AN ALTERNATIVE TARGET?

The Government has got itself into a muddle over targets for health care spending – a confusion it could easily have avoided and which was, especially given the scale of additional money for the NHS, unnecessary. But we have been here before. Labour's 1997 manifesto pledge card promised to reduce the number of people waiting for surgery by 100,000. Although they will almost certainly deliver on this, many pointed out at the time[6] that this was the wrong waiting-list target to set; waiting *time* was

more important, a view the Government has belatedly recognised in the *NHS Plan*.

There are of course good reasons for governments to set targets: they communicate intent and aspiration to the electorate; they provide a benchmark for measuring improvement; and they can help close the tax-and-spend loop by showing how taxpayers' money is being used. But there are also dangers with this approach. Among the political dangers is the setting of a target that will not be achieved.

If some fix on what we *ought* to be spending on health care is desired, then we would suggest that taking the EU average spend as a proportion of GDP (whether arithmetic or weighted mean) as a benchmark is too simplistic. Such a target fails to take account of how health care spending tends to change as GDP changes and also what the UK might realistically expect to spend given its wealth.

As Table 1 shows, in terms of wealth, the UK economy was the second largest in the EU in absolute terms (in 1998). However, we are not so rich in terms of GDP per head, ranking 10th out of 15. Striving to reach the spending levels of France and Germany may be inappropriate given our current wealth. In fact, there is a strong relationship between health care spending per head and the level of GDP per head. In general, as countries get richer they tend to spend proportionately more of their extra wealth on health care.

So, if we really want to compare ourselves with our EU neighbours (and in the case of health care spending this is perhaps debatable), then a more pertinent comparison should take account of what

Table 1: Total GDP and GDP per capita, EU countries 1998, US$PPP (purchasing power parities)

Country	Total GDP US$ppp	Rank	Country	Per capita GDP US$ppp	Rank
Germany	1,882,687	1	Luxembourg	37,613	1
UK	1,283,971	2	Denmark	25,687	2
France	1,278,310	3	Netherlands	24,119	3
Italy	1,214,328	4	Austria	23,872	4
Spain	679,442	5	Belgium	23,566	5
Netherlands	378,615	6	Germany	22,951	6
Belgium	240,446	7	Ireland	22,587	7
Austria	192,835	8	Finland	21,741	8
Sweden	184,697	9	France	21,721	9
Portugal	157,543	10	UK	21,675	10
Greece	148,391	11	Italy	21,312	11
Denmark	136,166	12	Sweden	20,867	12
Finland	112,030	13	Spain	17,257	13
Ireland	83,685	14	Portugal	15,787	14
Luxembourg	16,042	15	Greece	14,095	15

Figure 2: Projected health care spending per head and GDP per head, EU countries, 2006

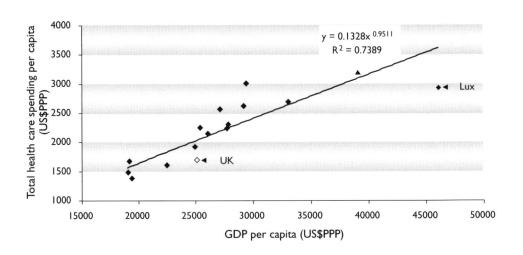

$$y = 0.1328x^{0.9511}$$
$$R^2 = 0.7389$$

we as a nation can afford to spend on health care.

Using linear projections of GDP and health spend per head (based again on OECD data) for the years 1960–99 to project GDP and health care spend per head to 2006 allows the relationship between these two factors in 2006 for all EU countries to be estimated (see Figure 2). The statistical relationship suggests that around 74 per cent in the variation in per-capita health care spending is explained by variations in GDP per capita, and that a 10 per cent rise in GDP per head leads to a rise in health care spending per head of 9.5 per cent.

From Figure 2, it is clear that given the UK's estimated GDP per head in 2006, its estimated actual spending will be around 19 per cent lower than could be expected. Put another way, the projected actual spending on health care as a proportion of GDP is 7.94 per cent in 2006, while the expected level – given the UK's per capita wealth – is 9.5 per cent. Compared with the projected EU average spend on health care by 2006 of nearly 11 per cent (see Figure 1), this alternative target – based on what we expect the UK to be able to afford to spend on health care – does not seem so daunting.

The estimates and projections used to arrive at this alternative target are of course subject to uncertainty. We cannot be sure that future EU spending will exactly follow the course we have predicted. Nor can we be absolutely sure of other variables used, such as the level of GDP in the future. Moreover, international comparisons of the relationship between GDP per head and health care spending per head need to be treated carefully.[7] Nevertheless, our approach to setting a global spending

target for health care is less arbitrary and, we would argue, more supportable than the EU average spend, however calculated.

Finally, the key consideration for government is how the extra money allocated to health care would be spent. This requires a more detailed consideration of the breakdown of the UK spend, both the distribution between different health sectors (e.g. cancer care or dentistry), and changes in the quantity of care, quality of care and rewards to those doctors, nurses and others who look after our health.

REFERENCES

1. Appleby J, Boyle S. Blair's Billions: where will he find the money? BMJ 2000; 320: 865–67.
2. Towse A, Sussex J. Getting UK health care expenditure up to the European Union mean – what does that mean? BMJ 2000; 320: 640–42.
3. Kavalos P, Mossialos E. International comparisons of health care expenditure: any lessons for health policy? LSE Health discussion paper no. 3. London: LSE, 1999 (revision of 1996 paper).
4. HMT Press Release. A Modern NHS: Fairness for families and communities. 21 March 2000.
5. HMT Pre-Budget report. Cm 4917. London: The Stationery Office, November 2000.
6. Hamblin R, Boyle S, Harrison A. The supertanker's not for turning. Lancet 1997; 350: 1493.
7. Kavalos P, Mossialos E. International comparisons of health care expenditure: what we know and what we do not know. Journal of Health Services Research & Policy 1999; 4 (2): 121–25.

—